TAI CHI

MOVING

AT THE

SPEED OF

TRUTH

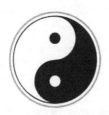

A NEW APPROACH
TO AN ANCIENT ART

W. B. BURT

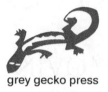

grey gecko press

Text © 2018 by William Broughton Burt

Design by Grey Gecko Press

All rights reserved. No part of this book may be reproduced or transmitted in any form or by any means, electronic or mechanical, including photocopying, recording or by any information storage and retrieval system, without permission in writing from the publisher.

This is a work of fiction. Names, characters, businesses, places, events, locales, and incidents are either the products of the author's imagination or used in a fictitious manner. Any resemblance to actual persons, living or dead, or actual events is purely coincidental.

Published by Grey Gecko Press.

www.greygeckopress.com

Printed in the United States of America

Library of Congress Cataloging-in-Publication Data
Burt, William Broughton
Tai chi: moving at the speed of truth / William Broughton Burt
Library of Congress Control Number:
ISBN 978-1-9457602-6-6
First Edition

To everyone who ever tried

to learn Tai Chi and gave up

THE ONE-PARAGRAPH PITCH

Please don't try to learn Tai Chi by rote memorization. That's the usual way, and it's a Confucian teaching device for a Confucian age. This book devotes over two hundred pages to fresh, original explanations of what Tai Chi is and how it works. As an educator, I've found that a principle-driven approach really softens the learning curve. Once we've absorbed the global principles of Tai Chi, the details more or less fall into place. Unfortunately, global information can be hard to come by in your usual Tai Chi class—which I'm not dissing. Really, there are some great teachers out there, and zillions of successful students. But modern Westerners need, uh, a little additional information. Confucians we are not. What we are is *busy*, and few of us are going to follow along obediently for three or four years in a program that's never been explained to us. You want my advice? Learn Tai Chi. Just however you can. It's that good. But do yourself a favor and read these pages first. You'll feel very empowered when you line up for that first lesson, and you'll stay loose and light all the way through the learning curve. That's important because you never reach the end of it. Tai Chi is all learning curve.

—*The Author*

THE ACTUAL INTRODUCTION

Shortly after beginning my adventures in Tai Chi in 1992, I went shopping for a few books to serve as an overview. Educators know that the global information needs to be there from the beginning, and I wasn't getting a lot of it, so I went in search of a few overview books on Tai Chi awareness and movement. There were no such books. Picture books, yes, but nothing that explained what it is we're doing in Tai Chi.

Clearly we're doing something.

The first time I saw Yang style Tai Chi performed in front of me, I knew exactly what I was seeing: I was looking at a technology. This was no quaint cultural exercise. Running beneath the choreography like an underground river were principles of human unfoldment that drew from the deepest of wellsprings. Immediately I was full of questions. Problem is, Tai Chi doesn't come with a lot of answers.

It didn't help that I lived in a rural cultural backwater, the American South, and this was before the advent of the internet. Local karate classes were the best I could do. I spent five years in Tang Soo Do and Shotokan classes while reading newsstand articles about the internal martial arts and dreaming of someday meeting someone who could take me there.

Finally I struck gold in twenty-eight-year-old Cangming Yang, a very accomplished Tai Chi practitioner from Shanghai who was pursuing graduate studies in a nearby college town.

Cangming had no time for me—he was sleeping maybe three hours a night—but he was kind enough to make me a copy of a VHS video of himself performing Yang, Chen, and Sun style—with *stunning* grace and precision. Over the following year, I taught myself the Yang Twenty-Four and Hundred-Ten directly from the video, Cangming providing the occasional critique of my progress.

But I still lacked that overview, that conceptual wraparound that would give me some hope of guiding my own Tai Chi practice in lieu of classes. I peppered Cangming with questions, but his English wasn't up to it. Nor, I suspected, was his Mandarin. What I was slowly beginning to understand was that the Chinese themselves lack an explication of Tai Chi. "Sometimes," Cangming told me once, raising a forefinger and smiling distantly, "is very interesting."

In pursuit of *very interesting*, I eventually spent a year in China. Too bad I was working four teaching jobs. I managed to attend a few Yang style and Chen style classes, hoping to casually follow along from the rear of the class, but because I was a foreign, white professional I was seen as some kind of honored guest. Every time I showed the slightest hesitation, they would stop class and *run* to the rear to give me a highly embarrassing personal demonstration of the entire form. I stopped attending.

My personal vision of Tai Chi, wherever it had come from, was of an essentially principle-driven art based not on choreographical details, but on natural human processes. Tai Chi was human alchemy. It was an enlightenment practice—not that I was enlightened enough to know what that meant. It was certainly the most perplexing challenge I'd ever undertaken.

And to the Chinese? The Chinese see Tai Chi as an enjoyable group activity, a shared daily ritual, a cultural affirmation, and a lighthearted gesture toward good health and longevity. Tai Chi to the Chinese is a nice hour at the park. All of which speaks to the overall balance and wholeness of the Chinese personality. It was *I* who somehow couldn't hold his mouth right. At any rate, I soon abandoned asking questions. It was like interviewing Americans on the deeper, more *cathartic* aspects of church league softball.

A mature Taiwanese master I met along the way confided to me that Tai Chi was never the same after the 1949 Maoist takeover. The Chinese Communist Party first banned Tai Chi as anti-revolutionary superstition—then required every schoolchild to memorize a severely stripped-down version because China had no public healthcare system; the doctors who hadn't fled the country had been sent to the countryside for re-education.

It was prohibited on pain of death, I was told, to teach the original version of either Tai Chi or Qigong. (It remains risky to this day, as witness the missing thousands following the Falun Gong purge of the late 1990s.) It's exactly that stripped-down version of Tai Chi that is now the world's most widely practiced exercise. If the deeper aspects of this ancient art have become elusive, it's little wonder.

By the time I returned home from China, I was weary of the whole enterprise. I'd put in eleven years. I'd taught myself the long and short Yang style forms on both left and right sides and could talk about Tai Chi as intelligently (in English) as anyone I knew. And I was terrible! Stiff, awkward, robotic, straining—I'd come to Tai Chi in search of magic, and all I'd found was a broken wand.

I gave up.

Quitting Tai Chi turned out to be one of the smartest things I'd ever done. It meant clearing out all my baggage around Tai Chi, and there was a lot of it, beginning with my huge store of expectations and demands both of Tai Chi and of myself. It meant clearing out my head, which was jam-packed with overlapping and conflicting details and poetic concepts that were, well, inscrutable. All of that finally went, and when the last of it was gone, my practice came to me.

I hadn't given Tai Chi a thought in several months when one afternoon, feeling very stiff, I rose from my computer chair and my body said quite pointedly, "I want to move."

"Fine," I replied. "Move all you want."

An instant later, like a bird released from a cage, my body *flew* into motion. Astonished, I looked down and saw my body doing the kind of Tai Chi I'd only dreamed of doing. It wasn't a sequence I'd memorized. It wasn't a style or a school or an approach. It wasn't an underlying principle. It was a self-sung song of joy.

I realized that something very significant had happened. An intelligence had *emerged* in me. Now that "I" had given up on learning Tai Chi, another part of me, one that had known all along, gently took control.

The next day I found myself moving again.

What was emerging was a different kind of practice, or *non*-practice, as I was no longer wearing the Mandarin collar or practicing the usual scales. My movement sessions became active explorations, and never the same experiment twice. I was no longer directing my process but simply letting movement well up and express out in ways I found impossible to anticipate or evaluate.

Suddenly I was experiencing *so* many things, not the least of which was a continuous lowercase ecstasy by means of which information would suddenly appear in me. I'd know how a certain move wanted to be performed and why. I realized that certain principles I'd learned were actually aspects of a deeper one no one had told me about.

These understandings didn't occur in my head but floated up from my body, which suddenly basked in some kind of inexplicable nurturing that I instinctively knew to trust. It didn't matter whether my intellect could sign off on what I was getting. If anything, these dawnings were to be trusted *because* they weren't coming from my head. They were radiating from an illumined body.

Anyway, I haven't read a word about Tai Chi since that day in 2003, nor have I consulted a single video or instructor, nor likely will I ever again. Have I become a master? Very far from it. To this day, I trip over my own feet. There's a lot I'll never grasp about Tai Chi, but there's also a bottom line, and I'll tell you what it is. I came to this practice to discover the power to transform a life, and I've found it, and I know that anyone can.

Tai Chi is incredible. If there's a hole in your joy, my friend, if you feel somehow estranged from your own life, locked away in your head, distant from your own experience—don't miss Tai Chi! Find a class near your home, commit to a six-month trial period, attend as regularly as you can, and keep this book handy. You're going to need an overview book, preferably one written by a really slow learner who went through hell on earth to access this information.

That would be me.

We won't go into martial applications or traditional weapons here, or the usual numbered sequences. And no pictures—sorry. But each page in this book absolutely speaks to every style of Tai Chi and every move and every practitioner every moment. Hopefully it will stimulate a much needed conversation about what exactly we're doing in Tai Chi.

Clearly we're doing something.

—*William Broughton Burt*
March 2017, Buenos Aires

How to Use this Clever Material

Use this material however you'd like, but Tai Chi beginners will do well to start at the beginning where I've tried to station the most urgent points and terms. Still in all, learning is a highly personal process. Skip around as you wish.

Here's an example of what I'm talking about. Let's say we're curious about investigating the ninth principle, The Circle. We add some circular shapes and motions to what we're doing and see how that feels. What's it like to be circular rather than angular? Give yourself several minutes to steep in one mode then the other. Then, while keeping Principle Nine active, start working with Principle Ten. Or Twenty-Three—wherever your curiosity lies.

See how many bowls you can keep spinning, how many of Tai Chi's principles you can activate at the same time. To the extent that we can activate them all, the result will be Tai Chi even if we don't know a single traditional posture. That's the power of the principles.

I encourage you to revisit each chapter periodically, as the learning curve is actually a spiral that returns again and again to the same lessons on higher levels. Scribble notes in the margins. Spill tea on crucial pages. Make a mess of this book and a diamond of your practice.

Insofar as general recommendations:

If you're intent on cultivating a meaningful movement practice, and you are, feather a really nice nest for yourself. Create a space. Going to classes is great, doing Tai Chi at the park or at the seashore is wonderful, but if you want this stuff to become a part of your life, it needs to become a part of your home.

How big a space? An eight-foot square (two sheets of plywood) is enough. If you're intent on doing numbered sequences, you'll need more room than that. Personally, I work with a snowflake pattern, facing each direction in turn, which requires very little space. If, for now, you have to shove the living room sofa aside—we all do what we can. Just try to work on a level surface and breathe good air.

Really try to work outdoors, my friend. It's important to breathe actual outdoor air, and not just for the oxygen content. Outdoor air is brimming with seasonal scents and pollens and pheromones and countless environmental cues that the body understands and processes on very deep levels. Then of course, there's *chi*, or life force energy, which tends to go stagnant inside buildings. As we'll see, chi is really important in Tai Chi, and we want to connect with as much of it as possible. So we practice in nature whenever we can.

If the air quality is poor where you live, practice early in the morning when pollutants are at their lowest and chi at its highest. Failing that, invite some broad-leaf houseplants into your indoor space, and make things as sunny and tidy as possible, and close the windows during the hours of highest pollution levels.

Better yet, move.

You may have found that big-city air gets you by just fine. But we're no longer interested in getting by just fine. We're aspiring to something very high here.

A few worthy details:

You might consider installing a good mirror where you practice. Tai Chi has both inner and outer aspects, and each informs the other. Without a mirror, you may develop the bad habit (as I did) of constantly bending forward to check the alignment of the feet. No. We want a consistently straight, tall posture in our Tai Chi. Get a mirror.

Video can be a great reality check if you've the stomach. I video-taped myself at the end of each of my first five years, recorded end-to-end on the same cassette, and I found that video log to be invaluable. Everyone is different, of course, and if we're really insecure about our bodies, we're probably better off skipping the video for now.

In general, let's not get too caught up in evaluating our progress. You and I are in no position to evaluate much of anything, okay? Our part is to show up, and show up again, and show up yet again. With each session, we're drawing imperceptibly closer to the sweet spot in our practice. We can't force our way there. We can't analyze our way there. We *can* move a little each day with awareness. That's our daily goal. So we keep a light touch. We're always alert to ways we can improve, but we aren't obsessing. You know what success in Tai Chi finally comes down to?

Being too dumb to quit.

Or, in my case, being too dumb to stay quit. Either way, just show up and pay attention, and I promise you fireworks and trumpet fanfares on the day when you least expect them.

What time of day is best for your movement practice? As mentioned, mornings are generally recommended. The air's good, we're fresh from sleep, and we want to set the proper tone for the day. But any time of day is fine, as long as we're not working on a full stomach.

You'll encounter a lot of *nevers* in Tai Chi. Never practice after eating or meditating. Never practice during an electrical storm. Never practice facing this cardinal direction or that one. Never practice in jewelry or a wristwatch. Never practice in shoes with synthetic soles. The list goes on and on. Listen, I've practiced Tai Chi every way there is, including drunk, and it's all good. Experiment. Find your own way.

Do intend to practice for at least fifteen consecutive minutes each day. Twenty is better, and sixty better still. But our daily goal is fifteen consecutive minutes of moving with full awareness.

When you miss a day or two of practice, don't obsess. We all miss days. Just look forward to your next session. Picture yourself there in your personal Tai Chi space, moving contentedly. Keep the energy light and positive, and a rhythm will develop that pulls you into its sway.

You'll probably want to keep a notepad handy. Intriguing ideas come to me when I'm moving. Before a practice session, I may look over the previous day's scribbles for a reminder of what I'm currently exploring. Select a nice notebook and keep your favorite pen right beside it—and a steaming cup of tea. Find small ways to invest in what you're doing.

Finally, and this may go without saying, if you don't have a Tai Chi teacher, you might consider finding one. The reason I never joined a class: there was no class available. If you are more fortunate, visit the studio and sample the ambiance. Does everyone look happy? Does the class start on time? Is the bathroom clean? Are your feelings positive in that space?

You won't find perfection anywhere, nor do you need it. Just go in with a humble attitude and soak up everything you can. Come a few minutes early and sweep the floor or tidy the bathroom. Bring fresh flowers. Contribute, and learn whatever you can, and when the time comes to move on, leave on good terms with everyone.

Don't show up at all unless you're willing to commit to at least six months of humble receptiveness. And don't quit without notifying the instructor and thanking him or her sincerely. Present a small gift, nicely wrapped, to cement what should be a lifelong relationship. In China, they say a teacher for a day is a parent for a lifetime.

You're not a joiner? Fine. Use this book as your guide and start moving.

What do I mean by "moving"? I mean stir about. Use dance music if that gets you going. If your Tai Chi starts out looking a bit like salsa, it starts out looking a bit like salsa. My salsa started out looking a bit like Tai Chi. Just use the principles in this book to inform what you're doing, and what you're doing will deepen in a hurry.

Again, work under a teacher if you can. Teachers and classmates provide pointers and encouragement, plus you're working with postures and sequences that have been around for a long time and have accumulated positive energy. Too, there's something called *direct transmission*, which means it's helpful just to hang in the presence of a really arrived practitioner, someone much farther along than yourself. You're entraining to that person's energy.

Finally, if you are a Tai Chi instructor, please consider presenting these forty-nine principles to your students. Every learner needs a conceptual overview, and you need a structured way of presenting one, or the results are going to be patchy. The last thing we want is for our students to feel outside their practice looking in.

Of course, many of the principles here describe not only Tai Chi but many other very worthy investigations into human potential such as acting and dance and yoga and the hard martial arts and various forms of meditation.

Whatever your focus, welcome to the book. There's room here for everyone.

PART ONE:
ATTAINING THE VIEW

A good pencil sketch captures the essence of a scene while leaving out many of the details. In the same way, this first group of principles sketches in the essentials of a good, deep movement practice. By activating each in how we're moving, we can go very deep, very fast.

The term *attain the view* comes from an old Tibetan Buddhist injunction concerning seated meditation. The first order of business, it's said, is to attain an expanded inner view by focusing on the bright spaciousness underlying form. At first, "bright spaciousness" is just another mental construct, but in time meditators perceive an actual field and are able to place their awareness there.

We're looking for that same kind of cognitive shift in our Tai Chi because that's where the juice is. If you're a martial artist, that's where you encounter the incredible power of chi. If you're ill, that's where you find your agency for self-healing. If you're interested in personal growth, that's where you encounter the power to transform a life. It lies in that cognitive shift where mental constructs give way to fields of information. There really *is* a bright spaciousness underlying form, and we've yet to come online as human beings until we've encountered that luminescence and opened it out in ourselves.

In Part One, we'll talk a lot about posture, which we'll learn is crucial to consciousness. We'll learn that different realities come into view as a result of different arrangements of the body. (Consider a TV antenna. One that's rusted, bent out of shape, and listing to one side is unlikely to bring in a very clear picture. Just so, when our bodies are neglected, misaligned, or stove-up, we don't get the picture in life. It's necessary to make adjustments in the array, and Tai Chi is exactly that process.)

Okay, we're about to open our very first principle of Tai Chi awareness and movement. A little drumroll would be nice, as this principle is so singularly important that we need to absorb it completely before we so much as glance at the others.

1. EIGHTY PERCENT EFFORT

In Tai Chi, we never strain
for a physical effect or a cognitive one.

Not long ago, there was an experiment involving the Tarahumara Indians of northern Mexico. The Tarahumara are famous for their ability to run for hours and even days on end, so researchers wired up a few of them and put them on treadmills in order to uncover their secret. At one point, the subjects were told to run really hard for a short interval, hard enough to create oxygen debt—and the Tarahumara wouldn't do it. They agreed to do it. They tried to do it. But in the end, they couldn't because abusing the body was outside their frame of reference.

Frustrated, the researchers packed up and went home, apparently none the wiser. The Tarahumara had revealed their *secret*, but the researchers had been intent on finding some kind of physical anomaly. There is no physical anomaly. There's just an understanding that life is a marathon. You abuse the body, you don't finish.

Tai Chi is about going Tarahumara. No matter the task of the moment, whether it's how high we kick, or how low we dip, or how many minutes we practice, we never go beyond eighty percent of what we're presently capable of doing. We sense where that limit is, and we don't go near it.

When I first encountered this idea, it floored me because I'd been a competitive athlete and a karate practitioner, and all I'd ever heard was a hundred percent effort, unless it was a hundred-ten. Once I heard a hundred-fifteen.

Now it's *eighty*? Really?

Really. When I lived in China, I was struck by the Chinese version of exercise. The Chinese seldom bother to change clothes or shoes but just step outside each morning and repeat a few simple whole-body movements, whether Tai Chi or Qigong or calisthenics or something else, and after a half-hour or so they're back to their day. No warm-up, no cool-down, no shower, no big deal.

By Western standards, that's not much of a workout. But they do it *every day* and, needless to say, the fitness and wellness levels of the Chinese far exceed those of the West. Here, the credo is overdo it or don't do it at all.

In the West, exercise is mind-over-matter. An unstinting mind forces a reluctant and comfort-craving body forward into good health. The mind may become smug about this, ignoring the body's cries for rest and referring to tidy charts and schedules for every detail of one's exercise program. The mind remains totally in charge of the process and—guess what? That whole attitude has to go out the window before we can even sniff Tai Chi.

In our movement practice, what we're learning to do is deemphasize the will of the mind in favor of the native wisdom and regenerative genius of the body. That's so important I'm going to say it again. In Tai Chi, what we're learning to do is deemphasize the will of the mind in favor of the native wisdom and regenerative genius of the body. That means, if today we feel drowsy, or gimpy, or bone-tired, or whatever it is, we respect that. We do less.

I know that's anathema in the West. Production is everything, right? Square that jaw. Throw that chest out. Hup, two, three—which is exactly why our health stinks. That's why we're so dazed we're staring extinction in the eyes and don't even care.

Globally, personally, however you want to look at it, *right here* is where the solution begins, here in our movement space, doing less for fifteen minutes each day. We guide the body through eighty percent of what it feels up to just now—and stop, still fresh. And probably quite a bit less drowsy, or gimpy, or whatever it was.

Let's be really clear on this. We are *not* talking about whiffing our workout. We're talking about something far more important than a workout or a hundred workouts. We're talking about reclaiming the body. We're talking about activating our deep organism.

Once the body emerges from its daze of chronic exhaustion, it becomes astonishingly transparent. Suddenly we're viewing a whole other landscape. We absolutely see a different world, but first the body has to recuperate from what we've been putting it through, and that can only begin by loosening the screws and learning to listen and respond to what the body has to say.

Tai Chi is about being the tortoise and knowing we're the tortoise. Our game is entirely different from that of the young heroes down at the gym. You know the type: world champs at twenty, finished by thirty, fat by forty. By age fifty, some of those guys are walking with a cane because they've totally trashed their bodies for the sake of being heroes for a brief moment of time. That's the hare, and we've no interest in his game.

It doesn't surprise me to encounter students with old sports injuries. What surprises me is the number of old *ballet* injuries I see. People may not even know that their shoulder problems, or their back problems, or their hip problems, go back to the unnatural postures they were forced into as young ballerinas.

I really don't know what we're thinking as a society when our most promising kids, the ones most gifted and passionate about moving, are the very ones shunted off to highly competitive and time-limited movement practices that leave them impaired for life.

I've yet to meet anyone with an old Tai Chi injury.

We've talked about the hare. Let me give you an example of the tortoise. Shanghai Master Ma Yue Liang, who lived to be ninety-six, was still practicing Tai Chi the final week of his life, and here's the thing. He was *better* at ninety-six than at eighty-six, or fifty-six, or thirty-six.

That's the tortoise: not very impressive in the beginning. Maybe still unimpressive ten or twelve years in. Fine. Not a problem. We're working on something, you and I. We're going ever deeper into a process whose implications are unimaginable. Only gradually does it dawn that, not only have we changed over the years, the whole world is different because of what we're doing.

That's our game. That's the program. To follow in Master Ma's light footsteps, which we can do, because all we need is time, and there's plenty of it. Tai Chi keeps the body going. This is a practice that absolutely knows and respects the design of the body.

Let's loosen the screws, people. Let's especially loosen them for the kids. Nobody needs to become a trophy cow for their parents. What young people need is to be guided into health-enhancing movement practices that deepen and broaden with the years. Once we're able to see that in terms of the kids, maybe we'll be willing to see it in terms of ourselves. You and I are ecstatic creatures, not production units. I should say that twice, but I'll let you re-read it. Until our lives reflect that truth in their every aspect, we're still in death mode. We're still part of a very ugly global problem.

The way we become part of the solution is, we personally cease to strain. We let the adrenaline drain from our bloodstream, and we let our minds run clear, and we become transparent to the truth of our situation. Then right action flows naturally.

Eighty percent effort applies equally to our altruism. Yes, we want to become everything we're capable of being, but first we have to be less than that, and effectively. I know that, globally speaking, it's late in the day if we want to save our world and our species, but the first thing that has to go is desperation.

What does that mean in terms of our Tai Chi? It means we're always *lightly* focused on straightening out the one thousand details of our posture and so on—but we're not pushing the river. We're *present with* our developmental processes. That turns out to be more than enough.

Same thing cognitively. We're highly interested in exploring our inner impressions in Tai Chi, and we're always leaning slightly in the direction of noticing a little more, realizing a little more, but any kind of straining "frightens away the fawn," to borrow a phrase from Tantra. It sets us back because we've banished the one creature—I call it "the deep organism"—capable of delivering us unto actual magic, actual transformation. By whatever name, there really is a highly advanced intelligence dwelling in each of us, and Tai Chi is that creature's process of stirring awake.

2. DROP DOWN

*In Tai Chi, we drop the
locus of perception into the body.*

The first order of business in Tai Chi is to get out of our heads. Doing Tai Chi from the head is impossible. I would know because I spent a lot of years trying. Like most Westerners, I'd been locked inside my head since first grade and had no idea there was an alternative.

There's an alternative.

In Tai Chi, we drop the point of awareness, *the locus of perception* it's called, from the head and diffuse it into the body. Why? Because you and I do not live in the world. We live in our ideas about the world, and that's a pity because the intellect is incapable of experiencing meaning or pleasure. If we want to experience either, it's necessary to step outside the box of thought.

In Tai Chi we spend fifteen minutes a day experiencing life in the raw. Afterward we're free to step back into our customary ideas, but when we do we're likely to discover that some of them fit and some don't. Beliefs, we learn, are frames to peer out through. Some are at times helpful, but frames are invariably restrictive because we can only see what fits inside our frames.

What made Einstein so smart? Was it the nifty frames of belief he was looking out through? No, it was his ability to remove his frames altogether and see the world in a childlike manner. That's what we do in Tai Chi. We spend a little time each day standing outside everything we know about the world.

And so enter reality.

What we're learning to do in Tai Chi is *feel* the world. I think it was Yang Cheng Fu, the man called the father of modern Tai Chi, who said, "The central issue in Tai Chi is feeling." I couldn't agree more.

Intermediate students, please take note. No matter how correctly you're performing the movements of Tai Chi, if you're not feeling anything, you're not doing anything.

Let's all of us take note. We can work really hard in our movement practice, we can bring such athleticism and grace to our Tai Chi that we win a boatload of trophies and attract a thousand students, we can learn to move almost exactly like our instructor and become a pillar of our lineage—and guess what? If we're not feeling anything, we're not doing anything. And feeling begins with getting out of our heads.

How do we go about doing that? Moving the locus of perception from the head to the body? First we find it. The simplest way to discover where the attention is, is to close our eyes and ask ourselves where exactly *we* are. Where in the body do we peer out from? Most of us discover ourselves in our heads, right at the center of the forebrain. Why there? Because that's the seat of thought, and we've all been taught that thinking is the single most important thing we can do.

If we'd rather locate ourselves at the center of the chest, for example, we just place our curiosity there, and off we go. It feels a little like descending a single floor in an elevator. You feel a little lighter for a moment, and then you're there.

Are you in your chest now? Notice how the left ribcage feels, then the right, then come back to the center of your chest. Now try to gaze upward at your own head. Just send your curiosity there without actually going there, and you'll see it there above you. How does your head look from the perspective of your chest? From your heart?

If you don't quite accomplish these noticings on your first try, no worries. It'll come. Just practice dropping down at the beginning of each segment of your daily practice, and you'll soon get it. Just don't use too heavy a hand. To make it easy, keep it breezy.

The first time I succeeded in dropping down was quite a surprise to me. This was before I'd even begun Tai Chi. I was practicing Soto Zen, one tenet of which is to experience the breath from the perspective of the belly (*hara* in Japanese, *dan tien* in Chinese). That had always seemed a peculiar notion, but I persisted in trying till one day while sitting I was alarmed to find myself in my belly, looking out.

It only happened that one time and then for only a couple of minutes, but I absolutely perceived the world from that spot. It only takes one such experience to know that "self" (which Buddhism says doesn't exist to begin with) is just a way of talking about the attention and where it chooses to dwell.

Listen, if there's anything more empowering than learning how to manage the attention, I don't know what it is. Functionally speaking, it's like this:

On your computer screen, where can you work? There's one place and one place only: where the cursor is. In your life, too, you can only accomplish something where the attention is. On the computer screen, how do you locate the cursor where you want it? You manipulate the mouse (using my old-fashioned computer, anyway). It's the same in your life. You move the point of attention by applying your curiosity.

Where did I put my pencil? As soon as the question arises, your attention is on the move, tracking the pencil. *Why hasn't Sandra answered my email?* Immediately your attention is on Sandra and the nuances of the last time you met.

The point is, we can let our focus drift aimlessly or we can put it where we want it. When we're doing Tai Chi, we want it diffused throughout the body, uncritically receiving information from any and every direction.

So, at the beginning of every session, and preferably at the beginning of each sequence, we witness our locus of perception dropping down into the body and connecting to what the body is seeing. Then we feel our connectedness expand in every direction till nothing is left out. In Tai Chi, we do this with eyes open and deemphasized. We're looking through the eyes of the body now, not the eyes of the head. Once we're practiced at this, we can drop down anytime anywhere in a matter of two or three seconds.

What do I mean by looking through the eyes of the body? Well, it's probably different for everyone, but when I drop down I find myself at the center of a landscape that's felt as much as seen. It's as though I'm noticing, with my inner gaze unfocused, every detail of an enormous multi-dimensional display that extends in every direction. I'm catching sight of ghostly geometric figures of various hues. I'm viewing complex energy architectures at every side. I'm tripping on the massive scale of everything. I'm feeling my effortless connection to each part of it.

When I'm seeing what my body sees, quite interestingly, everything I'm sensing is simultaneously sensing *me*. I feel the press of its intelligence. I feel the warmth of its good will. The only thing I don't feel is the need to ask questions. What's to ask? Suddenly it's all a simple matter of observation.

At first we find it easier to catch sight of what the body sees when our eyes are closed. What we want to develop in our Tai Chi is the ability to view the inner landscape with eyes open and softly focused on a real or imagined horizon. Once we've deemphasized the outer vision, the inner vision lights up and we realize that each of our one trillion cells is conscious, is in effect a fully functioning eye. Steering with our curiosity, we're able to blend our awareness with the awareness of all those one trillion cells. Our experience stream and theirs then flows as a single river.

When I first began dropping down, one thing I noticed was the peculiar sensation of blood draining from my head. It was like someone had pulled a plug. Only then did I know just how much energy is expended in the thought process. The moment we switch off active thought, that huge swell of blood can be directed elsewhere—to better uses, one assumes, than our usual enterprises of fretting, grousing, and speculating.

"But," you say, "if we're pulling blood from the brain, doesn't that mean we're getting dumber?"

Actually we're experiencing greater cognitive clarity. (I almost said "mental clarity," but those two words should never occur in the same sentence. *Mental* means we're engaging the thought process. It means we're up in the linguistic part of the brain, gazing out through its various frames of belief, which is exactly where we don't want to be. So, *cognitive* clarity.)

When we drop down, you and I are exiting linguistics and entering experience. We're no longer riding around in our thought-mobile in hot pursuit of linguistic truth. We're just *out* there, naked as the day we were born, radically opened up and paying soft attention. What we find is there's no need to pursue truth at all because it's coming at us from every direction, constantly registering to our finer senses.

What we're doing in Tai Chi is becoming more and more sensitized to those finer senses. We're activating a whole other sentience. If, as Claude Debussy has said, music is the space between the notes, intelligence may well turn out to be the space between the thoughts.

Obviously, there are moments when we need to balance the checkbook or make a dental appointment, so we do need to pop into our heads for a short time every now and then—but really, how often do those moments occur? I think you'll discover, as I have, that our lives seldom require active thought.

And we're not talking about shutting down the thought process altogether. We're just sidebarring it. As I go about my Tai Chi, my intellect is still streaming its customary commentary and I'm completely aware of what it's saying. The difference is, I'm no longer fear-induced to hang on its every word. I'm not sucked in by its attention-seeking behavior.

Our Tai Chi is teaching us another way of seeing and being. From now on, whether we're doing Tai Chi or some other activity, we're increasingly plugged into our *vast* array of sensory inputs.

Our thoughts are still streaming and we're free to "click on" a given thought, based upon its merits, and see where it may lead.

I very often click on a thought, even during Tai Chi practice. The difference is, you and I are no longer trading entirely in thoughts, leaping from one to the next as though there's no other place to stand. We've ceased being duped by the intellect that it alone has the answers, when in fact it doesn't have even one piece of credible information.

I say that because intellectual information is abstracted, deduced from something else, which too was probably deduced from some other thought. It's a book about a book about a book. Why, when we need information, do we so automatically go to the intellect when every other part of ourselves is connected in real time to the truth fields?

That's the question our practice poses each day.

What your and my Tai Chi is saying to us is: see how it feels to *feel* your way through life rather than worry your way forward. As you and I spend less time in the lonely haunts of the mind, we may find ourselves more connected to those around us and to our own intuition. We may feel more alert and curious than since we were children. We're experiencing life through the bright glow of the body now, rather than through the mind's dark lens.

We may discover that the body is always in a state of grace and enjoyment. We may find that we have to think in order to summon our lifelong anxiety or depression. Or, we may find ourselves face to face with emotional issues we've never allowed ourselves to fully experience. It's all to the good because we're becoming ever more present in our lives, and our lives are becoming ever more bitingly poetic.

3. Unhurriedness

*In Tai Chi, we move slowly enough
to notice every detail of our experience.*

I heard about a study done at the National Zoo in Washington, D.C. They wanted to know how long the average patron remained at a given exhibit, say the monkey cage, before moving on. What would be your guess? Two minutes? Five?

Ten seconds.

We begin this chapter at the National Zoo because it brings forward an important point, namely: the fast pace of modern life is a myth. The pace of life is determined by how fast we're moving, not the other way around. There's no one at the National Zoo herding us along with cattle prods. We're doing this to ourselves.

Tai Chi is a great way to undo all that nasty doing. Just a few minutes of moving unhurriedly each day is enough to remind ourselves that we have an alternative. Interestingly, the more we learn to slow down, the more we see into our internal processes and discover the hard knot of impatience and intolerance at our center.

I say, you and I are always hurrying ahead to the next moment because this one rarely suits us. Most of us dwell in a state of agitated suspension, longing to touch down in reality yet insistent that it first meet our standards. I can't imagine a more tragic penchant because this sets us apart from our own lives, placing us in a dead zone beyond reach of the simplest pleasure.

I think we perversely enjoy that little knot of impatience. It gives us something to gather ourselves around. Most of us end up cultivating our own brand of dissatisfaction, just as back in the sixties we each chose our own angry brand of cigarette. We opted for *edge* rather than repose because it was more available.

Still today we find ourselves in a hurried, harried, sardonic mindset fueled by trendy coffees and newspaper headlines and aggressive workouts at the gym. We go around collecting compliments on our non-stop energy level, and you know what? We're living our lives at the depth of a water-bug. We're making frantic designs on the surface of things, never achieving the least depth.

Personally, I rarely experience a moment of hurry anymore. I may occasionally glance at my watch and decide to move a bit more efficiently. But hurry? No. There's a difference, and the difference is whether or not we're loading fear.

You and I learn very early in our lives how to load fear, and not by accident. As small children late for school, we hear the word *hurry* countless times, and we register the tone of alarm with which it's said. We pick up on the tense, adrenaline-charged body language that accompanies it. We aren't being dressed by our mom; we're being roughed up by her. It becomes abundantly clear that a real and present danger is very close at hand, and here we are being trussed up as soldiers to be thrown out there willy-nilly to deal with it.

It's from such repeated cues that we all come to believe that a dark cloud of incalculable and irreparable harm hangs just above our tiny heads. Otherwise, why would Mommy be ripping out hanks of hair with the brush? If, decades later, we still scuttle about each morning as though ravening animals were at our heels, it's because we still sense that dark cloud of disenfranchisement and ruin hanging above us.

Ironically, if we're in fact running late and would like to advance somewhat more efficiently, the least helpful thing we can possibly do is load fear into our bodies. Fear makes us rigid, so now we're fighting ourselves, taking smaller and smaller herky-jerky steps, all the while struggling to accomplish them in more rapid succession. I'm sure we must look very comical in this state, like toys wound too tight.

Deciding to walk a bit more efficiently, on the other hand, is a choice like any other. We glance at the watch, decide we'd rather arrive earlier than now appears likely, and so, without tensing ourselves in the least, we stretch out our stride, covering more ground with the same number of steps. We're *gliding*, loose as a goose, enjoying the sights and scents of the moment just as before. We arrive at our appointment not only earlier but also in a relaxed frame of mind, instead of red-faced and cross-eyed, huffing, and cursing our delays.

Never hurry again. Make this promise to yourself and keep it.

How do we ensure that we keep such a promise? Our daily Tai Chi practice is how. That's where and when we install this new, saner way of being. We simply slow down and notice how we feel about that. Very probably, we're irritated at how slowly we have to move. We're vexedly thinking ahead to the next move, and to the end of our practice session, and to our plans for the rest of the day. So, we just *see* that.

Seeing is always our starting point. Noticing. The moment we notice something, it begins to change. So each time we find ourselves there-and-then instead of here-and-now, we simply see that and let it fall away.

Exactly how slowly are we supposed to do Tai Chi?

There is no correct pace in Tai Chi. We just make sure we're moving slowly enough to track all the details of our experience. That usually means we're moving pretty darn slow. Ultimately, forcing ourselves to move slowly is little better than forcing ourselves to move quickly. Both are forms of hurry because they're imposed by the mind on the body. What we're learning to do in Tai Chi is open a space of permission wherein the body can show us how it wishes to move.

Until that makes sense to you, experiment with various tempos. A quicker pace is good from time to time, as we can see how our bodies generate momentum for the next move. A brisk pace shows us how movement connects to movement. A slower pace, meanwhile, allows for more focus and more complete arrival in the moment, which is crucial to successful Tai Chi.

And then there's super slow motion, which takes us into quantum time.

Quantum time? Absolutely.

It's possible to slow ourselves to the point where time stops and maybe even flows a bit backward. Time is a personal experience, after all. Highly subjective, highly elastic. Some say highly non-existent. What we learn in Tai Chi is, the slower we go—if we're able to remain loose and soft—the more tiny increments open up in our awareness. Our experience stream breaks up into more and more discrete packets. It's like someone's printing them up.

Here's an example of what I'm talking about. If we're asked to raise our left arm, and we're agreeable, the experience initially registers as having two stations: before the arm is raised and after it's raised. The 'tween scarcely registers at all. Like when we're commuting to work, the 'tween is a blur in our experience because our focus is on points A and B.

If we now repeat the act of raising our arm, only with a bit more attention, we may discover that the arm *in motion* feels more interesting than either the before or the after. Now we're inhabiting three zones of experience: point A, the 'tween, and point B. After a year or two practicing Tai Chi, we're probably noticing and inhabiting a half-dozen or more increments within every movement, each with its own bouquet of nuances, each of them a complete experience.

After a decade of Tai Chi, maybe we're inhabiting two dozen, or three dozen mini-experiences per move, each of them at *least* as spacious and interesting as the two or three zones of experience we started out with. A stopwatch may tell us that our Fair Maiden Works at Shuttles occupies an insignificant span of time, yet our experience may be so rich and detailed that it registers as a lengthy, poignant adventure with various twists and turns and an ironic ending.

So, what *was* the duration of the move?

What's the length of a knit muffler? Seriously, if you were to hold a knit muffler lightly in your two hands, what would its length be? Four feet maybe? Now, enlisting the help of a friend, pull gently at each end of the muffler, stretching it till the holes are more apparent than the yarn. Now it's quite a bit longer because it's practically all holes. It's the same in Tai Chi, only we fall *through* those holes, through the spaces between the notes, and arrive at something that defies explication. That's quantum time. That's tiny increments. That's Tai Chi, and the only way you'll ever know what I'm talking about is to go there.

As our practice deepens, we find that points A and B pretty much fall away. We're living in the 'tween. Which is a good thing, actually, as reality has neither points A nor B.

Quantum physics aside, all we're really talking about is slowing ourselves down and noticing how we feel. You don't have to make it any more complicated than that.

So, how do you feel? If you're a beginner, you're probably feeling nervous and unsteady. Wonderful. That's where everyone starts. Now it's about patience and persistence. It's about coaxing ourselves into moving a little more slowly—without tensing up—and noticing how that feels. We're inching our way patiently toward the foreground-background reversal that transforms awareness and lives. That reversal absolutely comes. Never doubt it.

Incidentally, I decided to use the phrase *Moving at the Speed of Truth* in the title of this book because when I first began to feel chi, I found that it moved at a certain speed. When, for instance, I separated my hands and sent chi from one hand to the other (we'll get to that), I noticed there was a wait time of one or two seconds before the chi arrived at the other hand. Chi doesn't seem to be in much of a hurry, or that's been my experience.

Years later, I found information itself to be in motion. Truth is not stationary. Just as water maintains its purity only by moving, so does truth. You can't stop it, bottle it, and store it (as we attempt to do in books!) without truth degenerating into dogma. *True* truth is in a perpetual state of becoming, moving at roughly the same pace as chi.

An odd notion, I suppose, but it made perfect sense when I began to feel that pace and blend with it. Just as a swimmer can match the current of a river and blend with it, and perhaps feel for a moment that he knows what the river knows.

4. RELAXATION

The process of Tai Chi is largely one of discovering and releasing tensions in the body.

A bronze temple bell may make a very lovely sound, but if our arms are clamped tightly around that bell, all it can do is *doink*. In the same way, the body cannot radiate its self-joy and self-wisdom until we've learned to release the grip of tension that holds it mute.

This chapter is about how to achieve really deep relaxation in Tai Chi, but first we need to talk about why that's even important. Relaxation is about two hundred times more important than I once supposed, so let's talk.

Our last principle, Unhurriedness, said we should move slowly enough to notice all the details of what we're doing. The current principle says we can't do that without becoming really, really soft because those details register in the inner depths of the body. If those inner depths are rigid, we're that muted temple bell. We're just *doink*-ing.

Imagine, if you will, that you and I are composed of not just one, but a vast inner constellation of bells (quantum physicists say "strings," as in violin strings—same idea). What if each of our bones, each of our organs, each of our one trillion cells, were tiny temple bells carefully tooled to sound specific tones?

Now imagine having no tension anywhere in the body, nothing clamping down on all those bells. Imagine them all ringing out freely, creating lush harmonies and counter-melodies and overtones, all of it blending perfectly with an even grander music of the spheres that goes out and out forever.

Now stop imagining and start noticing because that's the story. That's your and my reality, but we won't know it as long as we're tight. We'll never know joy as long as we're tight, nor will we ever know our place in the scheme of things because, again, where those truths register is in the inner depths of the body.

As we know, bells ring in resonance with whatever sounds are passing through. They are receivers and repeaters passing along the information that's in the air. What if we saw the whole human organism in that same light? Every part of us is vibratory in nature, right? We all know that. Thus, when we're completely relaxed, every part of us is ringing with the truth of the moment.

We are *lit up* by the information passing through us, as was Pythagoras, to whom it was a completely audible sound he called "the music of the spheres." We're talking about not only something incredibly beautiful, but also rich with vital information about the Earth changes and the DNA changes and all the other things going on around and within us. We're *not* just talking about taking a few seconds to drop our shoulders.

Still, that's the starting point. Dropping our shoulders. We begin the process of relaxation by softening the obvious superficial muscles.

The Chinese call the initial phase of Tai Chi training *Remove the Toughness* because the body goes through an actual softening process that begins on the exterior then goes ever deeper. The Chinese say it takes a full year to remove the toughness. I say it takes as long as it takes. Meanwhile our health and well-being steadily improve because chi flows far more freely through a relaxed body. Actually that's a pretty big point because tension slows or blocks the movement of life force energy.

When we're tense, the thinking goes, our chi is sluggish and pools up, causing one part of the body to be too highly charged (*hot* in Ayurveda) while the spot just downstream is insufficiently charged (*cold*). This affects the joints, the glands, the organs, and everything else in the affected areas. Acupuncturists know how to intervene in such situations, but it's far better to undo the problem at cause, which is exactly what we do in Tai Chi.

In practice, relaxation comes down to two things: (1) noticing where we're tight right now and dropping it into the earth; and (2) discovering our deep tightness patterns and patiently working through them over time.

Let's start with number one. Where are you holding tension right now? Take a moment. If your shoulders are a little tight—that's most of us—notice that tension and release it into the earth. That means we exhale while imagining our tension melting away. It may help to raise them higher still, exaggerating the effect. Now drop your shoulders till they're just hanging on the connective tissues. The shoulders are a great place to start because we're unblocking the exact chi channels that nourish the heart, the lungs, the liver and the thymus, each of them hugely important to our health and well-being.

After the shoulders, we may notice that our abs are a little rigid. Notice and release. Then maybe it's the jaw. On and on. Much later we realize we're holding old emotional material deep in the body core. Same process. Notice and release.

One place we all tend to hold emotional material is the pelvic floor, a complex of muscles that webs the upper legs where they connect to the torso. We're talking about TAS, Tight-Ass Syndrome. We really want to be relaxed in the pelvic floor because that's where the base chakra is, which is where our body exchanges energy with the earth. If we're shut down there, we're shut down everywhere. Again, bring the area into awareness. Especially with the deep tissues, we're bringing our personal darkness to the light.

I think we're all acquainted with the idea that biography becomes biology. What happens is, certain parts of our body attract unresolved emotional material, and over time those areas contract and harden. The muscles and connective tissues may shorten until the joints can no longer return to their original positions. This leads to a chain of misalignments as the body attempts to adjust itself, and now pain can show up absolutely anywhere.

If you're experiencing pain, here's what the Chinese say. Move it away. Move that part of the body while intentionally relaxing it, and it will draw healing to itself. When we gently move any troubled part of the body, what we're saying to the deep organism is: *This place is important. Let's get it healed.* And the body gets it healed.

If you have a really resistant shoulder or hip or whatever it is, you may want to drop down to the floor and give it special attention. I call this *floor work*. While not part of Tai Chi per se, floor work has been invaluable to me. All we're doing is using the floor to help us isolate a tight place so we can coax it into deep-releasing. That's really hard to do on your feet because the muscles are "on duty." When we drop down to the floor, we can position ourselves so the tight area is unneeded. Now it can feel its way toward complete release. It helps to use our hands to gently probe that area and find the center of the contraction.

Now we "breathe there." We vibrate the area with our hands while projecting a mental image of spaciousness. It's a Tai Chi process, meaning we use subtlety and suggestion rather than confrontation and force. We're gently coaxing our fearful tissues into lengthening and releasing. If the area is holding old emotional material, we'll have to go back to the same area again and again because the body tends to gravitate back to its habitual patterns. It's a process.

Floor work, incidentally, is an example of what I call *sister practices*. Sometimes we achieve more by coming at a problem from a slightly different angle. I've pursued many sister practices over the years: Authentic Movement, Trance Dance, Healing Touch, Reiki, method acting, Holotropic Breathwork, and others. Each has shown me something about my movement practice.

As we progress in our Tai Chi, we discover how many fine degrees of relaxation are available to us. It's like our recent conversation about tiny increments of time. At first we may believe there are only two grades of relaxation to speak of: tight and loose. Over time, we come to know the many variables and subtleties at work within the organism. We each have an internal weather system with end-less variations and not-infrequent storms. Seasons pass through our bodies, and we increasingly learn how those seasons correspond to the outer events coursing through our lives, and vice versa.

Unlike external weather, though, our internal weather is some-thing we can do something about. Anytime we wish, we can choose to drop our tension into the earth, and open up our breath, and soft-ly rise in height, and come into proper focus as human beings. We can become a very different creature. As we continue to grow in our practice, we discover there are infinite increments of presence and pleasure available, fed along by infinite degrees of relaxation that de-liver us to ever more astonishing fields of nourishment and delight.

As far as I know, this process has no end point. Logically, I sup-pose it should. Once you've dropped your tension, you're done, right?

Well, all I can go by is what I've experienced. For me relaxation is a free-fall state. There's no end point. The softening sensation con-tinues and continues, opening and opening unto greater and greater fields of novel experience.

Imagine dropping a stone into a clear, shallow pool. You expect the stone to stop falling when it hits bottom—only in the present case, the stone penetrates the bottom and continues to fall, and you with it, experiencing its every dizzying moment of tumbling descent. I say, real Tai Chi begins at the point where that stone penetrates the sandy bottom.

It never stops falling.

5. OPEN AWARENESS

Our awareness is open and nonselective
in Tai Chi, receiving everything equally.

Tai Chi is about noticing. We'll visit this important truth now and again throughout our explorations, but here we focus entirely on the business of noticing because most of us do it wrong. Very few if any of us have been taught how to use our senses. In fact, we are widely discouraged from using them at all except when crossing a street. The rest of the time we're supposed to overwrite our experience stream with linguistic information—what we call *thought*.

And when we need some important piece of data, what do we do? Run to the nearest bookstore, newsstand, or net cafe. Information and linguistic information are no longer separate categories for us. There's no other kind of information out there. Right?

I suppose.

I was recently asked as part of a survey, what my preferred source of information was. It was a multiple-choice question. My options were television, radio, print, and the internet. I replied, "My eyes. I get up every morning and live in the world all day. I'm an eyewitness."

I think I failed the survey.

Listen, it's completely healthy to apprehend the world through our senses. We're designed that way. Take a look at your body. It's a mass of sensory inputs. Actually, every cell of the body is a sensory organ. Perhaps our whole purpose in life is just to open our many experience portals and witness this world straight-on and have it resonate in our every chamber. The problem is, we've largely forgotten how.

Tai Chi is a great, direct way of reacquiring the experience stream, of re-sensitizing ourselves to the simple, rich poetry of being. I say we really need that today because modern people are numb and looking for ways to get number. Drugs are just a small part of it. Look at today's movies. Look at what the kids are watching. *So* much stimulation. I can't even sit through the trailers, and I'm not just ranting here.

People gravitate toward what they need, and I understand that. There's a need for numbness in the world today, and people have every right to reach for what they need. I just don't want any. If you've made it this far into the book, you don't want any either.

In Tai Chi, what we're going for is *open awareness*, meaning we aren't deciding what is or isn't proper material for our noticing. We aren't blocking out. We aren't reaching. We aren't steering our experience toward "loving" or "spiritual" or anything of the kind. We're just opening all our many senses, including the ones we don't have names for. What comes in, comes in.

In my more poetic moments, I refer to this principle as Wind Through the Flute. In truth, you and I have certain things in common with a flute. We don't function very well without being open at both ends, to begin with. Only by letting the wind pass *out* can the wind pass in. So we're not grabbing hold of certain experiences any more than we're blocking others out. We're noticing how things feel as they pass through us. We're just a quietly alert real-time witness to what the experience stream bears.

Let me take a running start and try to say this.

In Tai Chi, we're constantly and uncritically receiving a self-refreshing overall *impression*, a stream of countless intermingling currents rich in color, bluster, and detail. Scents, regrets, leaf-chatter, the mood of the birds, the face of someone we spoke to earlier today, the crack in the pavement and the weed sprouting through it, our gimpy left knee, the purpose of life, the dull gaze of a passerby, the fire in our belly, the ant crossing before us. These things find us. We don't find them. All we do is hold ourselves so open, so vulnerable, that each impression hurts just a little.

Isn't that what we came here for? To hurt with the beauty of our lives?

No spinning allowed. If we honestly feel repugnance at something, it's our job to *be* that repugnance until the emotion fades. Of course the intellect will pop in and say, "Hold on, that's not spiritual enough. Quick, before someone notices, jump from repugnance to loving acceptance!"

But you and I aren't spinning anymore. We've given that up because an emotion is *exactly* what it is and can never be anything else. Feel it and it will consume itself quickly. Fight it and it's ours forever because it's lodged in the body. From now on, our work is in this moment, you and I. On the fly, no plan B, no straining, no filtering, no steering.

It's called honesty.

What exactly am I suggesting? I'm suggesting that you spend the rest of your life in an extended wild weekend love-affair with your senses, and that you do it with astonishing abandon and not the slightest sense of entitlement or ownership. Our experiences don't belong to us, after all. We just savor them as they pass through on their way to somewhere else. Wind through the flute.

6. Balanced on One Leg

*In Tai Chi, we always
have one leg solidly beneath us.*

In Tai Chi, the preponderance of the bodyweight is always resting on one leg. We're never fifty-fifty because fifty-fifty means we're immobile. So one leg supports us while the other holds our potential. That unweighted leg can very quickly become a step or a kick or a leg-sweep. What we're doing in Tai Chi is constantly stepping and shifting from leg to leg in a rhythmic sway. At a given moment we don't look like we're balancing on one leg, yet we are. We're at least sixty-forty (some teachers say seventy-thirty). That is, at least sixty percent of our bodyweight is resting on one leg.

There's never any muddy grey, is the thing. In the old books, this principle is referred to as Separation of Yin and Yang because we're making a very clear distinction. We have a *yang* (weighted, solid, masculine) leg and a *yin* (unweighted, empty, feminine) leg.

We're always separating and counterbalancing yin and yang in Tai Chi. If one hand is rising, the other is falling. If one body part is moving forward, another is pulling back. If one leg is set to the front, the other is stationed at the rear. Again, very clear separation. Look at the circle of two fishes. Do you see a grey fish?

How do we charge a battery? We attract all the positive to one side and all the negative to the other. Now we hold the two charges separate until we want to create a spark. That's separation of yin and yang. No muddy grey.

If we want to use that stored energy to turn a rotor, we constantly flip the polarity and the rotor turns. Likewise, in our Tai Chi we create strong contrast while regularly flipping the polarity—each time we take a step—which creates energy we're able to absorb into our organism.

I see the yin-yang circle as very literal. It's a schematic, actually, describing how energy is generated and moved in our particular reality. At first glance, the yin-yang circle is binary, meaning there's only black and white. But closer inspection reveals a third element: surrounding the two fishes is an all-encompassing outer circle called *Taiji*, the Grand Ultimate, from which our movement art takes its name. So in Tai Chi we're creating strong polarities and holding them in balance, which pops us out to the third perspective, that of infinity.

So it's very important to notice and sharpen the polarities in our Tai Chi. There's no end to this noticing and sharpening process, but there's definitely a place where we begin.

Observing the weighted and unweighted leg.

7. BEND THE KNEES

In Tai Chi, we never lock any
joint in the body, least of all the knees.

Why do we never lock our joints in Tai Chi? Because a locked joint, meaning one that's fully extended, is incapable of generating motion. Worse, it's just a fraction of an inch away from hyperextension and injury. We always want some play, some potential, in every joint of the body, which means we keep them reasonably near the center of their arc of swing. Nowhere is this more important than the knee.

What is the knee designed to do? To bend and unbend. Think of it as a door hinge. If you force a door open farther than it was meant to go, what happens? The screws start to pop out of the wood. It's the same when we lock our knees. We're using the entire weight of the body to hyperextend the joints.

If we habitually lock our knees when standing, that's a habit we need to unlearn. Locking the knees progressively stretches and lengthens the tissues along the rear of the legs without doing the same for the opposing tissues along the front. Over time, our legs begin to bow back grotesquely, forcing the hips to come ever more forward in compensation—which in turn leads to misalignment in the lower back, and on it goes until no part of the body is unaffected.

In our musculoskeletal system, everything affects everything. That's its design. It's a self-adjusting system. Our deep organism is always reading and responding, using the principle of complementary opposition to hold each body part in proper relation to the others. The body is incredibly adept at this, always reading and responding to whatever's going on, which is why every astronaut develops osteoporosis his or her first day in space.

Did you know that? As soon as the astronaut's body notices there's no gravity anymore, it says *okay, let's dissolve the skeleton.* Astronauts have to regularly communicate to the body that having bones is still part of the plan, which they communicate through—guess what?—a daily movement practice.

Your body, too, is constantly reading and adjusting to every change you make in your daily habits. At a given moment, the musculoskeletal system is conducting several concurrent waves of adjustments, and working out their interference patterns, and doing it all quite handsomely. Then why worry about it, you say? Why not just do as we please and let the body clean up the mess? Well, we can actually. It's called being young. That's what all young people do, and along about year forty a bill arrives in the mail.

Because the body is always listening to our behavior, our behavior becomes a language. Our daily Tai Chi session is nothing so much as a daily memorandum to the body that reads: *Dear body, all these joints and muscles and coordinating mechanisms are very much a part of the plan. We want it all tip-top starting right away. Thanks a lot. And the love handles are very nice, but any larger wouldn't work for me.* That's the message, and we're sharpening and reinforcing it every day of our lives. That's what drives the nail in.

Little taps. Lots of them.

People with joint pain really need to hear about "little taps." People in pain need every possible encouragement to move and keep moving because their doctors are warning them away from it. Doctors look at body parts like auto parts. When something wears out, it just wears out and that's it. All you can do is work around it as best you can or replace it with another one. You and I both know better than that.

Our joints are living things and vital parts of a living community with a will to thrive and the ability to adapt and heal, and they absolutely regenerate when given half a chance. Our best means of encouraging a compromised joint to regenerate is to use it gently and frequently. Little taps. Lots of them.

Again, if it hurts, move it. Every time a joint is used, the body feeds it, expediting blood and warmth and nutrients. When we don't use a joint, our memo reads: *Dear body, don't waste your time on this stupid joint because we're never going to use it again.*

Paul Lam says Tai Chi is the best joint therapy there is, and Paul Lam should know because he's a Tai Chi master and a rheumatoid arthritic. He's had it all his life. Lam is also a medical doctor, and Dr. Lam says every time we work a compromised joint, we may feel discomfort but we need to push gently forward anyway. Gently, meaning as low-impact and ergonomic as possible. That describes Tai Chi pretty well.

Dr. Lam participated in a very encouraging study (Song, Lee, Lam, and Bae, 2003) that showed a thirty-five percent improvement among arthritic women as the result of a twelve-week program of light Tai Chi. Yes, thirty-five percent—with zero ill effects reported by anyone.

So, knees slightly bent at all times. That's our new stance in life whether we're waiting in the check-out line, or yakking at a cocktail party, or using our computer. (I'm writing this standing up. Chairs kill.) Expect an awkward transition period. You may worry that your knees are going to buckle. They won't. You've just let the fine muscles and connective tissues around the knees become a little weak. Those tissues rehab in a hurry.

When I decided to go chair-free, I went through three weeks of sore legs and feet—but that was it. Three weeks and my legs were toned, my joints were solid, my bones were denser, everything had fully recuperated from sixty years in a chair. I'm telling you, the body is incredible.

Respect the process that is your body. And *really* respect your knees. If there's another joint in the body more crucial to personal freedom, I don't know what it is. Every time I see someone my age in a wheelchair, their legs withered and their skin turning grey, I feel just awful. Once the legs go, people—it pretty much all goes.

Notice, I said knees *slightly* bent. Remember the eighty-percent rule. Never make your legs tremble in exhaustion. Practically everyone past sixty does "high Tai Chi," meaning the knees are bent just a little. That's perfectly fine. Young Tai Chi practitioners tend to go for low stances because the dynamics are a lot more interesting down there—but that means separating the feet more (see Chapter Twenty-Two). Beginners should start out relatively high. You can drop down as your legs strengthen.

And again, we're talking about every joint in the body here, not just the knees. Some teachers want you to lock the elbow when you reach back in Brush Knee Push, for example. I don't get that at all. Tai Chi isn't about straight lines, and it certainly isn't about offering the opponent a free shot at breaking your arm. If that's the way your instructor teaches it—well, that's the way you need to learn it. But every time he or she isn't looking, do it the right way, okay?

Never lock a joint in Tai Chi.

8. BUDDHA BELLY, BUDDHA BREATH

In Tai Chi, the belly sags forward to
expand and contract freely with the breath.

It's impossible to talk about any body-mind practice without at some point speaking of the breath. Breathing is the only physical process that can be performed either consciously or unconsciously and so, it's said the breath bridges the gap between the conscious and the unconscious. And because the breath nourishes all the bodies, physical and etheric, it also bridges the gap between the limited and the unlimited selves. That's why a whole yogic science is devoted to the cultivation of the breath.

Really, every system of self-cultivation concerns itself with the proper use of breath. Even the most conventional physician will tell you that slowing and deepening the breath is our most direct means of calming and de-stressing the entire organism.

How do we work with the breath in Tai Chi?

We begin by wearing loose-fitting clothing. Tai Chi requires big-belly breathing, so no tight waistbands ever. Don't hesitate to wear something out of the ordinary. Uniforms are for uniminds. Personally, I find my Zen sitting robe perfect for Tai Chi. If it frees up the belly and allows for unrestricted movement, it's good garb for Tai Chi practice.

You and I tend to hold tension in the belly. I'm constantly reminding my students to release the belly forward, release the belly forward, because every one of us wants a flat stomach and very few of us have one. We also want to feel protected in this very vulnerable place, so we unconsciously hold in the gut. If you've developed this habit, undevelop it. You're constricting your lungs, which deprives the bloodstream of oxygen. You're also compromising the most important energy plexus of the body, the dan tien.

The dan tien (the Japanese say hara) lies roughly two fingers below the navel and one-third of the way into the body. According to the Chinese, the primary function of the *dan tien* is to store energy. It's our reserves. Practitioners of Qigong pay a lot of attention to the *dan tien*, charging it with energy each day. In Tai Chi, we're mostly just bringing the belly into our awareness and making sure it's not tight.

Actually, we want to encourage open breathing in all three sections of the lungs, upper, middle, and lower. In Traditional Chinese Medicine, those sections correspond to the organs of the upper, middle, and lower torso. If, for instance, the upper chest is constricted and our breathing is shallow in the upper reaches of the lungs, we're shortchanging the organs of the upper torso, including the heart, liver, and thymus, not to mention the lungs themselves.

Most people are more challenged in the lower part of the lungs, but we're each different. Investigate your own breathing habits and learn to animate the entire torso with each breath. Whole-body breathing. That's the objective.

Watch the way a baby breathes. Not only does the belly swell with each inhalation—the entire *baby* swells. The face, the arms, everything, seems to inflate and deflate with each breath. That's whole-body breathing, and it's exactly what we want in our Tai Chi and in our lives. Shallow breathing means shallow thinking and languid living. You and I want to live fully, and feel fully, and that means first of all breathing fully.

Be aware, too, that there are three stages of the breath: in, out, and pause. The pause should be a natural part of our breathing rhythm, not a forced holding of the breath. Many spiritual teachings speak of the importance of living in the space between the breaths, an idea richly supported by the research of Constantin Pavlovich Buteyko. (Look into his work if you're dealing with asthma, emphysema, sleep apnea, or any other breathing issue.)

Some Tai Chi instructors are really strict about breathing and require students to master the breath before they so much as learn their first posture. Once you've got the breathing down, now you learn to move in concert with the breath. Usually that means inhaling when withdrawing from the opponent or expanding the posture, and exhaling when contacting the opponent or contracting the posture.

I say Tai Chi is complicated enough without going blue in the face. The proper moment to inhale is when your body asks for it. If you want to move in concert with the breath, fine, but don't try it the other way around. It may actually be the ultimate insanity to have the mind telling the body when and how to breathe.

Again, visit your nearest baby. Babies are completely uninterested in impressing anyone with their yogic mastery of breath, so they breathe very irregularly, even fitfully, and seem none the worse for it. When something fascinates a baby, he or she may cease breathing altogether for a long moment, suspending their awareness in the space between the breaths. Then a few exuberant pants, and he or she is on to something else. I sometimes find myself doing the same thing when I'm really focused on something.

And we all breathe irregularly when we're sleeping, which would seem to make it a natural inclination of the body, right?

Go easy. That's all I'm saying. Work with the breath however you'd like, and there's much we can do—but finally we have to accept that the body already knows how to breathe. It's been doing it a long time. Our part, as usual, is to get out of the way.

9. VERTICAL SPINE

*The spine is soft and
consistently vertical in Tai Chi.*

Posture is crucial to consciousness. Whether we're exploring Aikido, or yoga, or meditation, or Qigong or Tantra—if we're working on ourselves at all, we're encouraged to become very intentional about our posture, and that begins with the spine. Simply put, we want a soft yet consistently vertical spine in Tai Chi.

Consistently vertical. That means head above shoulders above hips.

At first, verticality requires work because most of us are accustomed to slouching—but verticality actually requires *less* work because a balanced load is a stable load, and the human head weighs something like eight pounds. Offset the head just an inch or two, and the body experiences wear and tear along its entire length. Yet we've all seen photos of third-world women balancing enormous loads on their heads with no strain at all.

(Take note, dentists, hairdressers, massage therapists, energy workers, and others who spend a lot of time hovering over clients. Keep your hips under you, okay? When you need to lower yourself a little, do so by spreading the feet and bending the knees, exactly as we do in Tai Chi.)

It's about being vertical.

In our Tai Chi practice, we need to be especially alert when we're stepping and pushing, as there's always a tendency to lean in the direction of the push. Likewise, when we pull the arms back, we're tempted to lean back. No, no, no. It's just the hips that shuttle back and forth. The shoulders remain directly above the hips, and the head remains directly above the shoulders. This requires really close monitoring during our first year of practice, so that's what we do. We monitor really closely.

I've mentioned using a mirror as a reality check, and I'll re-mention it here. Actually, best would be two or three mirrors set at angles to one another, like in old-fashioned dressing rooms. That shows us really clearly when and how we exit verticality.

Because of computers, most of us have a forward hook in the neck and upper spine, and we're the last to realize it because it can only be seen for what it is in profile. That's where the mirrors come in. Be prepared for a shock.

Laptops seem to be especially guilty of pulling the head forward and down. If you use a laptop at home, work out an ergonomic solution. You can buy a separate monitor to install at head height. As mentioned, you can develop a stand-up workstation. You can also set a timer to remind you to check the position of your head every fifteen minutes.

In fact, every time the alarm sounds, hit *save* and walk away from the computer for a half-minute, raising your arms in the air, expanding your chest and popping as many bones as you can. Your eyes meanwhile should be focused on something far away. We do great damage to ourselves whenever we park our bodies in one position, any position, for hours on end. (I also recommend grounding either your computer or your body electrically. Research grounding or earthing. It's very important.)

I really worry about kids and phones. It's becoming increasingly difficult to encounter a young person in any other posture but wrapped around his or her personal electronic device. This disturbs me on so many levels I don't know where to start, but the health of the neck and upper back certainly comes to mind. That forward hook means our uppermost dozen or so vertebrae are frozen in unnatural positions. But it's the rule now. A forward hook just means you're literate.

The good news is, if we're still breathing we can thaw those frozen vertebrae and coax them back to life. We can recover full verticality, but it means taking time and trouble, as in a daily Tai Chi practice. And be prepared for a little transitional soreness in the neck. When something wakes up, it hurts, okay? But it's important to persevere. Press gently forward.

If you want to really work on your verticality, look into a Tai Chi drill called Pushing Hands. I'll talk about Pushing Hands in Appendix Z at the end of the book. That appendix also has more on the importance of the spine in Tai Chi.

Now, your Tai Chi instructor may very well tell you to always remain vertical and then instruct you to bend *way* forward when doing certain moves such as Needle at Bottom of Sea. Personally, I choose to remain vertical throughout Needle, lowering my hips rather than my shoulders. At the very end, when the downward hand reaches its lowest point, I curl my neck and head forward for just a moment, then I'm back up. I see other practitioners really emphasizing that forward bend, even bringing the torso parallel to the ground, and I think *ooh* that's got to be tough on the lumbar.

Likewise, Snake Creeps Down has us bending way forward at one point, but again much of that can be expressed by lowering the hips. Or just don't go down so far. Tai Chi is not athletic competition, nor any other kind thereof.

Even bowing involves a forward bend. Again my advice is, go easy. I've found that if, before bowing, you raise the hips a little as the hands are rising to the chest, you can then drop the hips just as the head tips forward, and it creates the same effect. Find your own way.

Finally, a vertical spine is not a fused spine. Don't be a stiff. In Tai Chi we're all about properly aligning the spine, and generating movement from the spine, and rotating around a consistently vertical spine—but the spine *has to* be soft and rubbery (or alive, or springy, if that says it better).

We go further into the idea of a rubbery spine in the following chapter. Listen, it doesn't matter how many times I've grasped the monkey's ears or repulsed the sparrow. It doesn't matter how many sequences I've memorized. If my body isn't soft and undulating and alive, my practice is stillborn. I'm just some stiff out there waving his arms around.

10. Body as Seaweed

In Tai Chi, the body should be like
seaweed responding to each passing current.

Seaweed on the ocean floor is never still, yet it never makes a single move. Seaweed is moved-by. It's pure black fish, pure transparency. It seems the pleasure of seaweed is to become a visible aspect of something otherwise invisible. You and I are the same in our Tai Chi, always moving yet responding to an impetus beyond ourselves. We're moved-by.

On a purely physical level, this principle is about having a soft, undulating spine that communicates movement from the hips to the shoulders and vice versa. We want the whole body as soft and flowing as seaweed. No robots allowed. We want waves of motion passing through the body.

Actually, there's no other way to move but wavelike. Before you or I can take a single step, we first have to shift the bodyweight to one leg. The act of shifting tosses the hips, which sends a ripple up the spine, and if the spine is rubbery and alive, that ripple is conducted undiminished to the shoulders, which then toss the arms, which in turn toss the hands, and finally the fingers crack the whip.

We've got these cause-and-effect loops moving through us all the time, and in Tai Chi we're alert to them and conducting them very knowingly. We want to be dead-on with each wave of movement that's passing through us. We want each *just* as coherent in the fingers as it was in the lumbar. All this is happening in slow motion, of course, which means the conscious mind has to abet the process, so now each wave is passing through body *and* mind. One definition of Tai Chi is joining body and mind through movement.

Here's a good way to work with this principle, Body as Seaweed. Stand in front of a full-length mirror and watch as your body conducts waves at various speeds. Just let your body undulate and watch how waves pass up from the lower body and out through the shoulders and appendages. Raise your arms and the effect is enhanced.

Check whether the rising waves are able to continue undiminished through the arms and finally pass out through the fingertips. Now get two or more waves going at the same time, and watch them interplay.

If you don't think too much, it all works out beautifully.

Interestingly, at a given moment in our Tai Chi there may be several concurrent waves of movement passing through the body. Before one can express out through the fingers, another has already begun churning through the body. And other dynamics are at work, too, like the swiveling of our shoulders and the rising and falling of our arms, and these things generate eddies and swirls of their own— all of which is being exquisitely *heard* by the whole organism. So at a given moment, body and mind are conducting a set of dynamics so incalculably complex as to be unprecedented.

Nothing in isolation. That's what we're discovering here. Nothing in the body, nor anywhere else, ever occurs in isolation. The behavior of each shoulder, each elbow, each hand, is always a necessary link in a complex chain of cause and effect that goes all the way back to the Big Bang and all the way forward to the destiny of existence itself.

So, we're not just *schlepping* our hand somewhere because it's in the choreography. The hand is impelled there, exactly there, by a succession of movements in the body that began somewhere else, linking us back, and back, to the original impulse that set the worlds in motion. That's the real wave passing through us, and we can only know its origin and purpose (and so, ours) by blending with it.

What I'm learning from my Tai Chi is, until something has happened in my body it hasn't happened yet. In some pre-logical way, I understand that these passing impulses come to me for a reason. They come so that they can know themselves completely, and their self-knowing becomes mine, as well. Tai Chi is a service we do, but I have to leave that for you to discover on your own.

As we progress in our movement practice, as we become better at softening and noticing, one of the things we're surprised to discover is that the very air is churning with waves of impetus and information and passion and inspiration. Our movements then become extensions of those impulses. We find that the earth beneath our feet trembles with emotion, and our movements should express those emotions in real time.

When doing Tai Chi we're picking up all manner of impulses, and as they inform our movement they become *our* impulses, our stories, while never really belonging to us. As with those lovely plants on the ocean floor, our pleasure is to become a visible aspect of something otherwise invisible.

I say seaweed knows what the ocean knows. How? By blending so perfectly with its currents that it becomes indistinguishable from the ocean. Seaweed never thinks about what it's going to do next, yet it's never wrong and it's never an instant early or late. That's exactly Tai Chi.

Now I'd like you to imagine something.

Imagine for a moment that you're a sea plant that wakes up one morning just really stiff in the neck and upper back. Let's say you slept wrong. How do the passing currents feel to you now? I'll tell you how they feel. *Ouch.* Each passing current batters the parts of you that can't move freely, and eventually those parts either soften or break. That's you and me, folks. If we're stiff, the waves of information passing through us are, number one, completely unknown to us—we can't detect them at all—and two, they subtly batter us.

You know where structural problems occur in the body? Where it's too rigid to conduct waves of movement. Where the energy stops is where the injury occurs. Every time you and I take a step, especially on a hard surface, a subtle shock wave passes up through the tissues and bones until it reaches something that can't move. There the wave stops, and that body part absorbs all the energy as damage. Your hips tight? You get hip pain. Your lower back tight? You get lower-back pain. Structural health is *very* much related to how transparent we are to passing waves.

11. ARMS SPREAD, ELBOWS DOWN

In Tai Chi, the elbows are held
away from the body and pointed down.

This should be unambiguous enough. In Tai Chi, our elbows are held away from the ribcage, never touching it. The shoulder joints should form roughly a forty-five-degree angle with the upper body. This expands our personal space. We're giving ourselves breathing room.

We're also establishing a perimeter. In the martial arts, there's something called *making a circle*. If some pushy person is crowding us and we don't feel right about it, we can make a circle by lightly touching his chest with the back of our forearm. At the same time we're smiling and saying conciliatory things, but the message is nonetheless clear. You're close enough, okay?

People who practice Tai Chi as a martial art understand the importance of maintaining a little air between our torso and that of an aggressor. We do that with our arms.

We're also careful that our elbows point consistently *down* in Tai Chi, and this too goes back to issues of personal safety. When the elbows are oriented down, the upper arms cover and protect the ribcage. We're also preventing the elbow itself from being seized and controlled. Once an opponent seizes your elbow and forces it up—the fight's over. So, even when a posture requires raising our hand in Tai Chi, we want to keep that elbow anchored to the earth.

Except for the exceptions, that is. Many people make an exception for White Crane Spreads Wings and another for Fair Lady Works at Shuttles. In those postures, we're instructed to place the upward hand above our head, which leaves the ribcage and elbow, not to mention our cheese, very much out in the wind. If we don't like the way that feels—who could?—we find a way to finesse the details.

Go with what you feel. Personally, I feel a strong pang of unhappiness in my ribcage when my elbow has left the building. So I raise the elbow only very briefly, meanwhile raising and lowering the hips to enhance the overall effect. It's a compromise but a calculated one.

Let's be very clear that Tai Chi is a martial art. Maybe we don't see ourselves as pugilists. Maybe we're not expecting a literal punch in the ribs today. But some subtler form of abuse is very probably on its way, and we need to prepare for that. It's tough out there. You and I require daily practice in dealing gracefully with conflict and even actual attack. We need daily practice in how to establish a boundary and insist on it without becoming upset or exhausted.

In Tai Chi, we're loading a very *relaxed* brand of assertiveness into our bodies and walking it around until it's just how we carry ourselves. No aggression. No paranoia. Just alert and confident.

Specific to the elbow in Tai Chi, we're supposed to spread our elbows to the point where a hen's egg can fit into either armpit, yet not so wide that the egg falls to the ground. Should somebody get pushy, the idea is to redirect him without either egg being crushed.

This we do by shifting our bodyweight and rotating our hips so that we aren't there when the shove arrives. We've moved to the side. Meanwhile, one of our forearms is touching and monitoring the aggressor, and we become the completion of whatever move he initiates.

Dumbfounded, our aggressor sees the error of his ways, apologizes most fervently, and goes straight home. We go home, too, and soft-boil our eggs.

Finally, let's be quite sure that the elbow doesn't point out to the side. Roll that elbow down and under (monitor Single Whip especially). An *out* elbow is not only a breach in our defenses, it introduces muscular tension in the upper arm and shoulder, which we've no use for.

Let's also note that the downward elbows serve to ground the upper body to the earth. Upper and lower come into proper relation, which is important in Tai Chi. At the same time, we're holding the arms away from the body, which fluffs us out. We become a different visual statement.

Think about it. When our posture is pulled in and our elbows are held tight against our ribs, what kind of visual statement would you call that? What are we feeling? It's like when our arms are crossed protectively over the chest. We're radiating fear. We're circling the wagons. We're closing for business.

And when we expand ourselves out? Personally, when my arms are opened out, even at a moderate forty-five degrees, I feel very expanded. I'm making myself available to experience. I'm open for business. I'm living wide.

Which could be another definition of Tai Chi. Being grounded and centered yet living very wide. As wide as the horizon's horizon.

12. Airy Hands

*The hands are soft and responsive
in Tai Chi, with a little air separating the fingers.*

In Tai Chi we don't want tension or rigidity anywhere in the body, least of all in our exquisite hands. Beyond the aesthetic considerations, consider too the energy meridians that terminate in each fingertip. Each of our fingers serves as a little on/off switch that influences chi flow in the entire body. (A raised finger decreases flow through a meridian; a lowered one increases it.)

I know one master, the distinguished Dr. Yang Jwing Ming, who likes to lift his forefingers a little while simultaneously lowering the middle finger of each hand. This, he says, adjusts his chi flow in a way appropriate to his constitution. Meanwhile, he likes to hold his thumb tight against the side of the palm, with the thumb-knuckle touching. Another instructor I know extends his thumb out at nearly a ninety-degree angle. It looks like he's signaling for a turn. Why? Because it feels right to him.

Best reason in the world.

There's a whole metaphysical science called Mudras that deals with hand positions and their energetic attributes. For me, simpler is better and simplest best. In my Tai Chi, I'm just softening and opening everything in sight. With the hands, that means letting them relax into a natural cupped shape with a little air separating the fingers.

If a specific posture requires one hand to close in a fist or describe some other shape, fine. I just keep the hand as soft as possible while forming the required shape. In the case of a fist, that means I'm not entirely closing the hand but leaving a hollow space at the center, with thumb and forefinger lightly touching.

In general, I try not to reduce my hands to any one expression but let them do pretty much as they please.

As beginners, we tend to micro-manage our hands, and that's completely understandable. But here's the thing. We're building toward the moment when we can drop all the conscious controls and just let our hands fly. Once we've internalized the principles of how to properly organize and array the body, we can drop a great deal of conscious control and just turn the body loose. That's where we're headed, and it's a very good space indeed.

When the hands can become a child of the moment, they can be quite magical. They roll, they expand, they comb, they describe, they respond, they question. In our Tai Chi, you and I definitely want our hands to be loose and spacious and plugged into the raw impulses of the moment.

13. DISTANT GAZE

*In Tai Chi, the gaze is level and
softly focused on the real or imagined horizon.*

Tai Chi is done *eyes out, energy out.* Our head is up, meaning level, our gaze is raised, too meaning level, and our eyes are fearless, both giving and receiving. We're mixing it up with whatever and whomever is out there, be it the devil *and* his cross-eyed girlfriend. That's important for each of us to hear because most of us are in the habit of withdrawing from the presence of people we don't know, and even those we do. We go internal. We tip the head forward and pull in the gaze, and we're gone.

Not in Tai Chi, my friend.

Once we've made the mistake of giving in to our timidity and dropped our eyes and pulled in our energy, our boundaries shrink around us and reflect our negativity back at us until we're a negative feedback loop. We're a self-poisoned pool.

Let me tell you a story.

Back before I moved to the country, I used to meet students in a lovely old city park with root-tossed sidewalks and massive trees festooned with flowering vines and darting hummingbirds and butterflies and dragonflies. It was an actual paradise. Migratory birds dropped in regularly, making each season a different display, a different soundscape, a different string-ensemble of scents. *What* a place.

What a place this Earth is! For each of us, natural beauty is a required nutrient, and in Tai Chi we're mainlining the stuff. We're constantly turning in every direction, our eyes receiving and scanning into our deepest recesses every nuance of the environment. We're making the beauty around us a part of our cellular life. That's why it's so important to have our eyes lifted and actively *receiving* the world as we move.

These days I'm blessed to practice Tai Chi in my own private garden, which too is heaven at the very least, but I want to take us back to that root-tossed and *festooned* city park for a reason. It was there that I first came into possession of my eyes. Until one very singular moment in that very singular space, my eyes were a pair of fugitives darting here and there, never finding rest. Until then, they'd never felt secure enough in themselves to begin their great work of receiving the world.

Call it shyness. Call it cowardliness, but for nearly all my life, my eyes had been locked onto the pages of a book or some scrap of paper. On the rare occasions when I was caught in a situation with no linguistic materials at hand, I simply shut down. My eyes went dark, completely uninterested in the present situation. Why should they be? They were in the wrong place viewing the wrong things. I'd missed a turn along the way, or I'd boarded the wrong train, and now my rightful place in life was accessible only to the imagination. In effect, my eyes were the barred windows of a prison cell.

Then came a day in the city park when I was leading a couple of students through a sequence of Tai Chi moves. All at once, I noticed a preoccupied young woman in a blue jacket passing by. As she passed, she turned for a scant moment, less than half-curious, to observe us. I spent that same scant moment observing her observing us. Then she was gone. The experience lasted maybe three seconds.

I haven't been the same since.

Maybe you, like me, feel conspicuous doing Tai Chi in public. We *are* conspicuous. We're breaking all the unwritten rules of public comportment. We're being extraordinarily open and truthful and beautiful, and our energy is expanding in every direction, and people can't help but notice that. People may even be shocked by that. I've had the police show up and question me. I'm not kidding. Someone had called them.

On the other hand, it's only natural that we occasionally feel the impulse to *break out into Tai Chi* in a lovely outdoor setting, so there it is. We begin to move, and people give us a curious gawk, and it's usually fine.

It's also really interesting. What we're doing is so powerful that people sense it even before their eyes catch sight of us. They turn and they're like *oh there it is*. To the extent that we can weather that kind of scrutiny, to the extent that we can pull it off and be that naked and that beautiful in front of everyone—we're providing an incredible service. We're lighting up everything in sight. That's the way I look at it.

Then there are other moments when maybe we don't quite pull it off, when we let our fears shut us down. All of a sudden we're demonstrating all the wrong things. Maybe we're going through the motions, we're parting the horse's mane and all the rest of it, but we're not *doing the deal*. We're no longer open and including every living thing we see, and people sense that. People know the difference.

For years and years that's exactly where my Tai Chi was. Shut down. To an extent, I was shut down even when practicing alone. In public places, it was just that much worse, and *because* it was worse I was finally able to see that and decide to change.

With an assist from a young woman in a blue jacket.

The thing about Tai Chi is, we're noticing everything. Even despite ourselves, we're noticing, noticing. We're moving so unhurriedly and with such presence, there's really no place to hide. So every time I succumbed to my fears in public and shut myself down, I was immediately choking on negative energy and *longing* to open back out. I knew I was making everything worse by dropping my eyes because now I was imagining that people were mocking me when they very probably weren't.

Why the light finally came on for me that particular day, I can't say. I think I was just tired. Sometimes being tired helps us because we can't quite load all our usual horseshit. We're just not up to it. Plus, I may have felt somewhat bolstered by the presence of my two students. Whatever the reasons, at the precise moment when that young woman appeared in her blue jacket and her preoccupation and her half-curious gaze, I couldn't quite muster my usual paranoia. Instead there was a tiny tug of *curiosity*.

Who is this person? Why that particular look on her face? It was only a tiny tug, but somehow even that small scrap of curiosity made me invisible. I was able to return her gaze as though from a place of hiding. Then the young woman was gone, and I felt something unusual. It was like a key turning in a very old, rusty lock. Somehow in the rush of the moment I'd forgotten to worry and I'd not been punished for it, and something popped open.

For the remainder of that Tai Chi lesson in the park, I *relished* holding my gaze open, no matter who was within it, evil adolescents, construction workers, the devil himself, the cross-eyed girlfriend, it didn't matter. I included them and didn't care a fig whether they included me or not.

Again, I haven't been the same since.

So, eyes out, energy out. Giving and receiving. Gaze softly focused on the real or imagined horizon. Peripheral vision fully activated.

Yes, it's okay to blink. I'm always surprised when someone asks whether it's okay to blink our eyes in Tai Chi. Blinking is the body's way of cleaning and lubricating the eyes, and it also ties into mental processing. We don't need to micro-manage all that. As with the breath in Chapter Eight, the mind comes to the body for instruction in Tai Chi, not the other way around.

14. ELONGATE THE BODY

*In Tai Chi, we're consciously expanding
and lengthening every part of the body.*

Do this.

Place your two hands palms-down on a desktop. Line them up evenly, the fingertips of each hand extending forward equally. Now relax both hands and tell one of them to elongate. You're just saying to one of your hands, "Longer, longer," and imagining the hand lengthening in response to your suggestion. (Don't let the suggestion bleed over to your other hand. Separate them a bit and focus on just one.) Give the process thirty seconds or so, and see what results you get. I just did the experiment here at my desk. My results:

Length of time—five seconds

Amount of extension—half an inch

Maybe your results are more showy than mine, or maybe they're less so. But listen, if your hand elongates *at all*, we're onto something.

What we're onto is the body's amazing ability to expand and contract, and its even more amazing willingness to go along with the suggestions of the mind. In this chapter, we'll talk about the importance of having an expanded, elongated body, and we'll compare our method to the more conventional practice of stretching.

To begin with, and this is a little obscure but important, we may not generally think of our joints as being in either an expanded or contracted state. We tend to think more about arc of swing. If the arc is shorter in length than it should be (we can't kick very high), we may initiate a stretching program. But there's arc of swing and there's *degree of expansion.*

Maybe the reason we can't kick very high is that the femur (the thigh bone) is retracted into the hip socket. That happens when the soft tissues of a joint, any joint, tighten up and pull in. The result is a joint that's constricted at its center, not along its arc, thus our best efforts at stretching are going to meet with very limited success. Why? I'll give you two reasons.

First, we're not working at cause. When we're stretching, we're trying to solve a subtle internal problem in an aggressive external way, and that's not going to work very well. Secondly, contracted tissues *cannot be stretched.* We think we're stretching them because we see a temporary increase in our arc of swing. In fact, we're traumatizing those tissues, and our joint health is going to suffer as a result.

What? Stretching doesn't work? Then how do we expand contracted tissues? By releasing them. We use auto-suggestion and focused breathing and visualization, and we encourage the tissues to release their grip—and they do, usually in a matter of seconds. Remember? Half an inch in five seconds? And that was just a hand.

You wouldn't believe the things I've seen.

I'm not totally against stretching. After a joint has released, it's fine to do some light stretching. Never *before*, is the thing. When we attack any tight area of the body with an aggressive stretch, the tissues tighten even more in self-protection. It's called *the muscle spindle reflex.* We're working at cross-purposes with ourselves. The thing to remember is, the body is always listening. There's no need to shout.

In my karate years, I did all manner of devilment to myself with ill-considered stretching techniques. I had one of those stretching machines that forces your legs apart with a crank and a bicycle chain. It was monstrous. I would sit in that contraption for an hour at a time, reading a book and occasionally cranking my legs out a little wider. My body complained bitterly every step of the way, but "no pain, no gain," right? I have only one word for that kind of stretching now.

Rack.

In Tai Chi, we begin by viewing the body as a thoughtful, responsive being always to be approached with respect. If anything, we're dealing with an intelligence superior to our own, so if we want the body to soften and elongate, we just communicate that in the most direct language available, which is intention and visualization. We project an image of a loose, happy, open body whose joints are progressively expanding at their centers.

Immediately we feel the body soften and lengthen in response to our suggestion, which reinforces our projection, and now we're surfing a positive feedback loop. We fall deeper and deeper into that sensation, and magic happens. All that remains to be done is to walk the whole musculoskeletal system through eighty percent of its range of motion, and we're done.

It's called Tai Chi.

What we do in Tai Chi is see the whole body as constantly expanding, beginning with our first move. As with many of the principles in this book, it's a good idea to install a checkpoint early in our daily routine, in this case one that coincides with an expanding physical movement. Without a checkpoint, we're very likely to forget this subtle principle, and we definitely don't want to do that.

We want to see the spinal column lengthen, creating generous spaces among the vertebrae. Many people have pain issues due to a compressed spine, and they're told there's nothing to be done but cut and suture.

Again, the body's listening. There's no need to shout.

"Taller, taller, taller . . ." We simply whisper this to ourselves at the onset of our daily Tai Chi session and feel the expansion that occurs throughout the body. You tell me. What's better? Cutting or whispering?

Finally, it's important to consider that a persistently contracted joint is usually related to an emotional issue, and that issue may have to be dealt with before the joint permanently releases. In Appendix

Z, I go into detail about one such case, my own, and the three years of hard work that finally resulted in a permanent release in my chest area and a new lease on emotionality. We're not necessarily talking about a quick fix here. Still, I see release work as a *very* direct and powerful way to achieve healing on physical and emotional levels. It's what we do in Tai Chi.

Listen, how far we're able to go on this magical mystery tour of ours depends entirely on how profoundly we're able to soften and open the body. It's a long-term project that begins again each moment with our re-commitment to becoming incalculable, illimitable creatures. Creatures beyond even our own understanding.

15. THE CIRCLE

Tai Chi favors circular
shapes, movements, and themes.

Your and my ancestors noticed that birds and other animals construct their homes in a circular shape, and that all living things are influenced by moving circular shapes in the sky that depart and return along circular pathways. They saw that every natural cycle is a circle in the dimension of time. Every emergent culture has claimed the power of the circle for its pottery and basketry, its baked breads, its shelters and its community design.

Later it was understood that the Earth itself is circular, and furthermore spherical, meaning an infinite number of circles sharing a single center-point. Then it was learned that our planet has spherical brother and sister planets that describe circular orbits around a spherical Sun, which itself makes grand transits of the Milky Way galaxy, and on and on and on.

It's puzzling that modern man has developed such an intense relationship with straight lines and perpendiculars, which are completely synthetic, all but unknown in nature. The conquered nomadic peoples of the American West resisted moving into square houses until the end. They knew what it would do to them. (Now the question becomes: what might it do *for us* to return to circular living? I jot this question at dawn at a circular table at the center of my circular home, which has sheltered and prospered me for four years now. Personally I couldn't be happier with life outside the box.)

It's how we're designed, you know. As Leonardo famously illustrated, every joint in the human body is intended to describe broad circles through space. Thus, when our movements are circular rather than straight, we're blending back into our original design and thus our original impelling directive.

In your next movement session, switch back and forth between straight lines and curves. Notice how each feels, how each colors who you seem to be and what you seem to be about. When you're circular, what kind of creature are you, and what kind of cosmos do you live in? And when you're angular? We can choose which one to be, just as light chooses each moment whether it's particle or wave.

Personally I find sharp angles a little threatening, like a pair of scissors lying on a bed. Straight lines connote hurry. When we are straight, we're destination-oriented. The Chinese say that straight lines speed up the flow of chi, causing distortion and discomfort. No Chinese would live in a home at the end of a long straight road that points like a gun barrel at the front door. How could anyone find rest in a home like that? And what of our gridded cities, everything so rigidly boxy and line-of-fire? Everything in modern urban design and modern home design is guaranteed to stress you out.

"The curved line," said the architect Antoni Gaudi, "belongs to God." If that's the case, we humans might want to borrow it for a little while.

In Tai Chi we include the circle in everything we do and thus *are* included in the nature of things. We're mindful of avoiding sharp angles in our elbows, wrists, knuckles, and so on, softening everything into graceful curves. Our movements describe circles in space, and our sequences describe circular narratives in time, as we always end a Tai Chi sequence in the same spot, orientation, and posture where we began.

More grandly, a Tai Chi sequence is best seen as our own personal transit of the grand cycle of existence. We begin in stillness with our weight equally distributed, which symbolizes the original void, *Wu Chi*, the vast undifferentiated sea of potential that underlies form. In the beginning, we're told, nothing existed but Wu Chi. Then all at once, something specific popped out of all that formlessness. Our Tai Chi sequence reenacts that primordial moment when our bodyweight shifts to one foot.

Of course, that specific development gave rise to its opposite—which we can readily observe, as our weighted foot gives rise to an unweighted one. So now we have polarity, and we're off and running.

Our Tai Chi sequence goes on to express "the ten thousand things," meaning all the various configurations of yin and yang that constitute the world of form, before finally and neatly folding itself back into the two primordial opposites. At that poignant moment, we're back in our original spot with the bodyweight resting on one foot. Our final act is to return the bodyweight to the center.

Poof. We've vanished once more into Wu Chi. We've made the complete circuit from emptiness to form and back to emptiness. "And the end of all our exploring," notes T. S. Elliot, "will be to arrive where we started and know the place for the first time."

So here's the question. In our Tai Chi, do we symbolically reenact the first moment of creation, or do we *enact* it? When we close our stance at the end of the sequence, are we dramatizing the final moment of existence, or do we bear it on our tiny wings? Just how close at hand is the cosmic drama? Is it possible for you or me to stand even a hair's breadth away from birth and annihilation, ever? Doesn't that occur ceaselessly within us, thousands of cells dying each moment, thousands of others newly born, while all around us stars and entire galaxies are birthing and dying, the universe itself experiencing both its creation and its demise?

My observation is that it never stops for a moment. Consciousness is incapable of achieving separation from either the first instant of creation or the last. Or that's what my Tai Chi is telling me.

What does yours have to say?

16. LESS IS MORE

*In Tai Chi, the lesser
the force, the greater the power.*

Where I live in the high mountains, there's a long dry season. The wind blows the dust around until it becomes a homeopathic version of itself, lighter than helium. Try to sweep it up, and you're tasting it in your mouth.

Unless you do Tai Chi sweeping.

Being very clever, you and I know to hold the broom vertically and move it in a continuous, unhurried circular sway, never applying undue force. That gets the dust into the dustpan rather than into our lungs. Less, in the end, accomplishes more.

In our Tai Chi, we're very sensitive to this point. We aren't throwing our weight around. We aren't overpowering, or over-reacting, or over-committing, or any of those other overs that equate to under-paying attention.

We've talked a little about Pushing Hands. Pushing Hands demonstrates the futility of overpowering our opponent. He or she just fades to one side and uses our momentum to send us sprawling. If we catch ourselves over-committing and try to back out of the trap, that too sends us sprawling. We screw up every time we make a decision because deciding slows us down. It puts us one step behind the action, and we're easily beaten by an opponent who simply remains on center and responds to what's happening. In that sense, the principle Less is More is about not getting caught up in our own ideas, not being hoisted by our own petard.

Let's put the same idea slightly differently. It's not the use of brute force that's wrong in Tai Chi or in life. It's the use of *only* brute force. It's hitting the situation over the head with a big white fish when our Tai Chi is telling us to come from both sides of our nature, from our power and from our absence.

What does that mean exactly? First, if we're directing a push in a certain direction, we're pushing with everything we've got. We're pushing with our determination, we're pushing with our rage, we're pushing with our earlobes, we're pushing with our premolars and our grandmother and whatever's in the checking account—it all goes. Nothing held back. But we're pushing, as well, with our vast *emptiness*.

We're empty of hurry. We're empty of fear. We're empty of expectation. We are an alert, neutral animal observing a gesture that we, at the same moment, are totally committing to. It's when we dip equally into both of these deep wells, the solid and the empty, that we summon the Grand Ultimate. We bring in something whose power surpasses itself.

Nobody here is suggesting that we do anything halfway. We're not talking about a medium grey. Diluting our strength and our commitment is no solution to anything. When we say less is more, we mean we're mixing a very small amount of pure white fish with an enormous quantity of pure black fish. That's balance.

Look at homeopathic medicine. It's practically all empty space. A homeopathic remedy contains a very minute particle of the active ingredient, yet the medicine is perfectly balanced. Consider that a single lead weight calls on an extraordinary number of feathers. By their very natures, yang is highly condensed and yin very diffuse, so in Tai Chi we're mixing a *very* small amount of brute force with an extraordinary amount of emptiness. Note that the icon of the two fishes shows them equal in size, but that's not a depiction of ratio. It's a depiction of balance. If we were to depict ratio, all we'd see is black fish. The white would be too tiny to register.

Still, that tiny bit of masculine energy has to be there, and it has to be radical. We're totally buying in. All our passion and purpose is focused into this one gesture, and if we have to pay with our lives we're ready. We're ferociously ready. That's very pure white fish, and it's required. Either we bring that kind of commitment to our every moment in Tai Chi or we're wasting our time.

And then there's Madam Black.

How do we call in Madam Black? We leave open a space for her. In Tai Chi, we learn that the greater the space we leave unoccupied, the greater the presence of the mystery. So we're really committed, we're really strong, we're indomitable, and we're also leaving an enormous space open for the black fish.

In Tai Chi, we're receiving more than we're giving. We're listening more than we're speaking. We're being moved more than we're moving. We're putting a lot of air around whatever we're doing, especially whatever we're theorizing, because that keeps us alert and on center and responding to what's going on around us in real time.

We're coming from *both* the extremes in ourselves because that fires up an engine powerful enough to send the bad guy flying across the room and halfway through the drywall. That's how it works.

Let's just be very aware that, in Tai Chi, balance means mixing a very small amount of irresistible force with a very considerable amount of allowingness. Whether or not we become capable of sending someone crashing through the wall, we'll have learned the proper way to operate a broom.

[Author's note: This may be a good moment to reassure the reader that our constant commerce with the unknowable in Tai Chi has absolutely nothing to do with black magic or evil or any other such tepid bit of nonsense. The black fish has no qualities. Qualities of every kind emerge from the black fish, yes, but the moment they are knowable they've migrated to the other side.

The black fish is a doorway open to the night. Whether we are safer with that door open or closed isn't even a question because we're talking about the better part of what we are. We can't escape that. We can waste it. In Tai Chi we dance with the unknowable because it's the only dance there is. We do it because we are born dancers. And we do it because we are interested in the unlimited generative power of that which lies beyond common knowing.]

17. THE INNER GLOW

*In Tai Chi, we increasingly notice and
interact with a very bright inner luminosity.*

Tai Chi is most essentially a mystical practice, a means of sensitizing ourselves to the web of life that interconnects and sustains us. Tai Chi, too, is an alchemical practice because we are transformed by that deepening connection.

If you've never heard of the mystical/alchemical side of Tai Chi, it's because the subject was declared taboo in the 1950s. That's when the Chinese Communist Party began cleansing China of everything they saw as traditional, superstitious, or personally empowering. Something like ninety-five percent of Tai Chi wound up in the waste basket. Two generations later, it's hard to find anyone in China who's both willing and able to talk about the deeper aspects of Tai Chi.

Fortunately, as mentioned earlier, Tai Chi is holographic. All the information is contained in each of the parts, so the mystical/alchemical roots of Tai Chi are still there to be discovered by anyone who really wants to find them.

Here's a question for you.

If you were to close your eyes right now and send your awareness into your body, if you were to light up that whole inner space with your perception, what would you find? A beating heart hopefully. Maybe a little tightness in the shoulders. Maybe a dull ache in one place or another—and not a whole lot more. Or that's what our education has prepared us to believe. The body is a dumb-zone, a place of gurgling organs and random discomforts. One might even question whether heightened body awareness is a good thing. What could *the body* possibly contribute to the conversation?

To learn the answer, we have to go a little deeper. We have to send our awareness into the space underlying the body. Not into the flesh itself but into the multi-dimensional space upon which the body is written. There we discover something called subtle energy, or chi, or *prana*, or *orgone*, or the aura, or the consciousness field. It's been called a lot of things. I just say the inner glow.

Tai Chi is very much about subtle energy. We learn to feel it, and generate it, and move it, and enjoy it. The average Tai Chi practitioner becomes aware of chi in about the fourth year of practice, but it doesn't have to take that long. Most of my students experience chi in their first class.

Consider this your first class.

Take a moment now and hold your hands body-width apart, palms facing each other. You can do this standing or seated. Without giving it too much importance, begin to notice how the space between your palms might feel. Let it be a peripheral kind of thing. Don't stare directly at it. After half a minute or so, you may decide that you feel some kind of sensation in or between your palms. You may think of it as pressure or density or attraction or repulsion or any number of things. Maybe the flesh of your palms feels a little rubbery. Just be with whatever you're getting, even if it's nothing at all.

After a minute or two of peripheral noticing, begin to bring your hands very slowly together. Note any changes that occur at the edges of your perception. Once your hands are almost touching, begin moving them apart again. Finally let your hands drop to your sides.

How about it? Feel anything out of the ordinary? If so, congratulations. You've just "found your chi," as we Tai Chi insiders like to say. Your task now is to develop the ability to feel it at all times with eyes open.

No real impressions? No worries. Just return to this experiment once a week or so, preferably after a practice session. I promise that before long a breakthrough will occur.

What is chi? It's just the way the universe is wired. Most Tai Chi people talk about chi like it's wall current—just blind power. Which is true, and it's not true. On a certain level, chi is much like wall current. You can learn to sense it, you can interact with it, and you'd better learn to respect it or it can burn you down.

Case in point: Once at a weekend Tai Chi workshop, I had lunch with a woman who'd studied under a renowned master in New York. (One of the best things about weekend workshops is lunch because that's when you hear the *real* stories.) Because she was an advanced student, this woman's master sometimes used her in demonstrations. In one such demonstration, he was a bit distracted and accidently sent chi into her with a strike. The poor girl bounced off a wall and hit the floor unconscious. She woke up in a hospital bed. You only have to hear a couple of such stories to know that chi is, among other things, a devastating weapon.

My lone misadventure with chi was more comical than injurious. I'd read about a meditation technique that circulated chi in a very particular way. The book warned against using the technique when seated in a cross-legged position, but I thought, "Oh, what harm can it do?" So I crossed my legs and went to work.

About two minutes later, I began feeling really sick. Then an uncomfortable knot of energy began forming in my groin. In a panic, I reversed the technique for a couple of minutes then massaged my dan tien for a while, and I was fine. What did I learn? I learned not to toy with this stuff. There are details you can fudge, and there are details you can't fudge, and it requires a lot of study and experience to know the difference.

Turns out, there are many different kinds of chi. The Chinese recognize roughly three hundred fifty kinds. Some are like the wall-current variety described above, while others are of a higher thread-count.

All I can talk about are my own experiences. Aside from the above misadventure, all my encounters with subtle energy have been spiritual in nature, which is to say conscious, benevolent, and nurturing. When I tune into the inner glow, I come into the presence of an intelligence far superior to my own. That intelligence is aware of me, and meets me where I am, and fills me with inexplicable pleasure and knowing. Maybe it's just my dumb luck; maybe it's that the universe reflects back to us what we're putting out.

Maybe we just find what we're expecting to find. If we're expecting to encounter blind, brute force, we'll probably experience blind, brute force. I was coming from a different direction. Perhaps significantly, I was initiated into Reiki early in my Tai Chi journey, which attuned me to a range of frequencies many would call spiritual.

When I do Tai Chi and contemplate who the ancient Taoist masters were, I sense that their motivation was to draw from the deepest, purest wellsprings of truth and empowerment. I'm convinced they wanted to access the farthest reaches of human potential and push those limits out even farther. The word for that process is *alchemy*. To me, that's the heart of Tai Chi.

Of course you may find something entirely different, and neither of us has to be wrong for the other to be right. We all discover what we come to Tai Chi to find. For most of us, it's a way to take care of our bodies. Many of us come to Tai Chi for beauty's sake alone. Then there are the martial artists among us. I simply entered by a different door.

My own preference is to bask in the inner glow. That's what it seems to be for. Communion. Healing. Pleasure. Illumination. Evolution. I just hang in that rarified space, basking, diffusing my awareness into that amazing, brilliant luminescence that stretches as far as I can see. Each time I enter those pleasure fields, I marvel anew at the intelligence and goodwill and nurturing I encounter.

It seems totally clear to me that this is why we do Tai Chi. To re-inhabit our astonishingly connective nature and discover on the most personal of levels what the human experience is and where it can lead.

PART TWO:
GROUNDING OUR PRACTICE

In Part One we encountered a handful of concepts crucial to establishing a meaningful and transformative Tai Chi practice. In Part Two we ground those ideas into the earth. Remember the metaphor of the antenna? No antenna is properly installed until it's grounded by means of a copper stake driven into the earth.

This, we're told, drains off random electrical noise and provides a clearer signal. You and I, too, function far more effectively when properly grounded, and the following twenty-one principles of Tai Chi awareness and movement provide a means of driving that stake really, really deep.

18. Horse and Rider

In Tai Chi, the lower body is a horse,
the upper body a supple, responsive rider.

You may recall the mammoth Tai Chi study done by Emory University *et al* late in the last century. A fifteen-week period of moderate Tai Chi practice was shown to reduce falls in the elderly by a surprising forty-eight percent. Researchers scratched their heads and said the improvement was probably due to improved inner-ear function.

Nonsense.

The people in that study got off their asses once a day and strengthened their trunks and legs. I'm a senior myself, and I can tell you that old people don't just topple over. We get tripped up like everyone else, and we lack the lower-body strength and quickness to catch ourselves.

Let's get stronger in our trunk and legs. That's the message here. No more of this falling down business. In undeveloped regions of the world where people squat and sit on the ground as a matter of course, you don't see seniors crashing down like loblolly pines and shattering their hips. Why? Because those people have *legs* under them. In the third world, fifteen weeks of Tai Chi practice would reduce falls in the elderly by what? Two percent? Five, tops? And you're telling me *forty-eight*? Only in America.

The Chinese say the lower body should describe a horse, and they're absolutely right. The lower body does all the serious work, all the heavy lifting, and that part of us needs to be rock solid. The older we get, the more urgent this becomes because when the legs go, it all goes.

The upper body, meanwhile, should be upright and loose like a skilled equestrian. I like this metaphor because the ideal rider is small and lithe and transparent to the movements of the horse below. A good rider becomes part of the horse because otherwise he or she gets beat the hell up. A poor rider gets off the horse at the end of the day hurting all over. Those of us who experience back, shoulder, or neck pain need to consider whether our upper bodies are responding to our lower bodies as they are designed to do.

Everything begins with the horse, but before we leave the subject of the rider, let's establish one important point. In the West, we define fitness by how rock-hard the upper body is. This applies especially to men, who want to be massive in the chest, shoulders, and neck. But for all of us, fit means hard, right?

No, it doesn't. If we're talking about the upper body, fit means soft. Fit even means small.

Ever seen a jockey up close? A jockey is a very small human. His job is not to overpower the horse but to get out of its way. Put a bulked-up muscle man on a horse, and you've got a horse lugging around a lot of dead weight. After a long day of riding, both horse and rider are going to need a good massage. Similarly, when we go to the weight room and add pounds of upper-body mass, we're adding dead weight, meaning mass that doesn't support itself and that doesn't move in concert with what's happening below. When upper and lower body disagree, there's trouble ahead for the lower back.

We want to *be* stronger, not look stronger. That means we work the postural muscles, the ones that hold the body up. We want mass that supports itself, not mass that has to be lugged around. I'm not saying stay out of the weight room. People over fifty have every reason to go to the weight room because their muscle mass is melting away with the passing years. I'm saying bodybuilding is wrongheaded unless you're working the lower body at least as hard as the upper—safely—and working on flexibility and whole-body movement along with bulking up.

One more caution about weightlifting, and we'll drop it. Our bodies are built on the concept of opposing muscle groups. You can't just work one side of your arms, for example, or legs or torso. You have to work the opposite side equally or you're distorting yourself and sooner or later you're going to encounter injury. Too, the various parts of the body are designed to be flexed from a variety of different angles, which is all but impossible to duplicate in the weight room.

If you're lifting a lot, you can't go from there to participating in a complex, vigorous sport without risking injury because you've created a Franken-body that's adapted itself to one environment only: the weight room.

Go easy. That's the advice here. If you lift, work as many muscle groups from as many angles as you can, and allow plenty of recovery time. Better, strengthen the body by doing what the body is designed to do, which begins with walking, which begins with getting out of the chair, which begins with realizing what the chair is doing to you.

Here's a nice study for you. Americans who sit for more than three hours a day die two years ahead of schedule. If you're watching TV while sitting, you die three and a half years ahead of schedule (Katzmarzyk, Lee, 2012).

I said goodbye to television four decades ago. Last year I cut chairs out of my life. There's still dinner with friends, of course, and rides in taxis, and so forth, but I no longer sit when at home. As mentioned, I have a stand-up workstation, and I've put a strap on my guitar so I can play standing up. My dulcimer, a lap instrument, is now installed at stand-up height, as is my musical keyboard. When I feel like resting, there's a big padded rug in the living room topped by a cotton blanket. I'm either up or I'm down. I don't mess with Mr. In Between.

My back loves me.

Fitness turns out to be a pretty simple matter. We're not talking about a moon shot here. Once we're out of the chair, we're half done.

The other half? We step outside and put one foot in front of the other. Not with weights strapped to our ankles. Not with little pink barbells in our hands. We walk *our* weight. We walk our own center of gravity. We let the body find its own exact measure.

And don't go near a treadmill. I'm sorry if you just bought the latest model. Treadmills are the equivalent of eating dog food. Have a little respect for yourself. Walk your weight and your center of gravity out in the fresh air and sunshine. Commune with the birds and the flowers for a while, and when you arrive at your destination, let it be a beautiful place to practice Tai Chi. And I don't want to hear: *oh* it would be wonderful if I lived in a place where I could walk outside, but—

Stop. I'm not listening. If you have the money in your pocket for a bus ticket, you're living where you live by choice. If war and plague erupted in your city, I think you'd find a way to get out of there. You'd grab your toothbrush and the hand of your loved one and you'd split. Well, this just in. There *is* war and plague in the city where you live, and the casualties are astronomical. Get out of there.

Again, it's really pretty simple. Live where life is good. Work the horse. Relax the rider. Squat from time to time—without weights on your shoulders—and occasionally sit or lie on the floor and rise back up.

I used to attend an acting class where we went to the floor for warm-up drills. Most of the students were in their fifties and sixties, which is not ancient, but they were totally lost the first time they had to find the floor. It was even worse when they had to get back up. The teacher had to go around and talk people up. *Turn onto your side. No, onto your side, like this. Now bring your knee forward. No, your knee. Watch me.* The good news is, a few weeks later those same people were different creatures entirely. They *flowed* down to the floor and back up. Their whole way of moving had changed, along with their attitudes.

I recommend a bit of floor work as part of any daily movement practice. Maybe that translates as a few yoga postures. Maybe it's a simple stretch or two. I know one man with back problems who rolls around on a wooden floor each day and swears by it. It's not so much what we do down there; it's mostly the going down and the rising back up. Once we're handy at doing that, we're less terrified of falling. We're also less likely to fall because we've strengthened that horse.

It's about the horse, people.

One specific note about lower-body fitness: most of us don't realize how frail and weak our ankles are. We may never think of our ankles at all until we "turn" an ankle, which can lead to a dangerous fall. Where I live, there are some really rough cobblestone streets, and turned ankles and falls are frequent among visitors. People who live here year-round develop strong, flexible ankles and seldom have a problem. How strong and flexible are your ankles?

We find out in a hurry when we begin doing Tai Chi because we're required to balance on one leg. Typically, our support ankle trembles and falters and we say, "Oh, I need to work on my balance." That's not your balance. That's your puny little ankle, and you're doing exactly the right thing for it.

If you wear high-topped shoes or lace-up boots, get rid of them. Or at least save them for a special challenge like a mountain hike or a visit to my cobbled town. Used every day, high-tops make your ankles progressively thinner and weaker, and nobody wants that.

Again, insofar as the upper body, it's not about strengthening so much as softening. The upper body is the rider, remember, so its well-being depends entirely on its suppleness.

When practicing Tai Chi, we want to be very aware of upper-body softness. We're aware of conveying successive waves of movement up the spine. Even the slightest lower-body movement should send a ripple up all the way to the top of the head. When we're walking, we want to be aware of softening and loosening with each step, of conveying those same waves. We're particularly aware of the sacrum and tailbone. It's important to have some wiggle in our walk. Every part of the body should be flowing with each step.

Sometimes this principle, Horse and Rider, is stated a little differently. You may hear the lower body likened to the trunk of a tree and the upper body to its branches. Same idea. The lower body should be like a tree trunk, swarthy and tenacious, grasping the earth so as not to be uprooted. The thin, pliant upper body, meanwhile, is like the tree's branches that surrender to the wind. Masculine below, feminine above. Everything working together by working differently.

19. THE ROOT

*In Tai Chi we cultivate a
very strong connection to the earth.*

Sometimes at Tai Chi demonstrations, an elderly master will challenge several young men to move him off his center. The crowd loves this stunt because the young men look comically inept, tugging and shoving in vain. The master, we're told, is unmovable because he has "sunk his chi," meaning he holds such a clear vision of his body's connection to the earth that the two are inseparable. I've no doubt that's true, but the master is also a master of body positioning.

He maintains such a low center of gravity and twists and contorts so expertly in response to each gambit that—well, how do you push what you can't find? So there's a metaphysical kind of grounding, and there's a physical grounding, too, and we need to understand both.

I think we all know what's meant by a grounded person. It's hard to mislead such a person because he or she is in solid touch with reality. In a crisis, a grounded person doesn't waste a lot of time running around in circles but goes straight to the solution.

And an ungrounded person? He or she is always in crisis mode, always late, always misplacing the car keys at the worst possible moment, and can't quite grasp a simple solution to anything.

We've all experienced moments when we've felt really grounded and intuitive. Maybe we're fresh from a week-long camping trip, and we come back to our routines feeling marvelously centered and alert. Decisions are effortless because there's always an obvious choice. Conversely, a shocking experience such as a burglary or an auto accident may suspend us in a bubble of bewilderment for weeks. Anyone can lose his or her grounding, and it's important to know how to get it back.

Tai Chi is how.

Question. What is the nearest planet in our solar system? When I ask this question, I'm always surprised how many people reply Mars or Venus. The nearest planet is called Earth. Look down. You'll find it there.

The Earth is not a concept. It's a ponderous reality, and to discover that, we need to escape our carpets and our concrete and our elaborate foot-wrappings and—dare I say it—touch the planet.

How long since you've placed a bare foot on the damp, naked earth? How long since you've drawn that magical sweet scent up through your bones? How long since your corporeal self has experienced direct contact with the elements of which it is composed?

I think that's important. If the body never touches anything but plastic, it feels alien and wrong. To relax into a sure understanding of itself, the body needs to experience the touch of its own kind. When the feet touch the earth, the body feels moving within its own architecture the familiar song of its origins. And it feels joy.

So whenever we can, you and I need to practice Tai Chi barefoot on the naked ground. If that's too scary for us, our shoes should be simple, light affairs made from natural materials. No neoprene soles, no arch support, no heel. The sole should be flexible, and the fit should be loose.

Tai Chi is generally practiced in shoes because it comes from a shoe culture, just as karate is practiced shoeless because it originates from a barefoot culture. History is history. God bless every bit of it, but what we need to be talking about is *our* practice, and the only question that matters is what's right for me?

Personally, I want to be as primal as possible during my fifteen minutes a day. I want to be everything my most distant ancestors were. I want to know what they knew. For me, that adds up to working barefoot on raked builders' sand. If there was a rain last night, it's wet. If the sun's on it, it's warm. If I forgot to cover it last night, there's a memo from the neighbor's cat. It is what it is and, because of that, I am what I am.

I won't push this idea because it freaks some people out completely. And working barefoot is more difficult. Our base is narrower, so we're unsteady. We're bringing a lot more foot joints into play, and those joints may not have been used in a long time, so yes, we're suddenly teetering like beginners. But listen, our feet are coming alive and flexing in ways they can scarcely remember.

Our toes are actively and separately grabbing the earth, and we're getting all our reflexology points worked (especially if there are pebbles mixed into the sand). We're conducting electricity up from the earth, and we're feeling more alive in our fifteen minutes than we're likely to feel all the rest of the day. But, again, it's just a suggestion.

If our aim is to establish a profound connection to the earth, it becomes really important how the foot contacts the ground, the floor, whatever. The yang, or weighted, foot needs to be as flat as possible with the toes fanned out. That foot, weighted evenly front-to-back and side-to-side, becomes our ear pressed to the earth. It's listening, absorbing every faintest message. The center of the sole, meanwhile, is making solid contact as well, which stimulates an acupuncture point called the Bubbling Well.

Which brings us to the whole topic of stance, doesn't it? Stance is hugely important in the martial arts, so let's talk about it.

First of all, a good stance requires setting the feet widely enough for good stability. We never put ourselves on a tightrope. In general, we're setting the feet hip-width apart, meaning the outer edge of each foot is directly beneath the outermost point of the hips.

Likewise, we need to be *long* enough in our stance for good front-rear stability. For high Tai Chi, that usually means heel/toe (the rear of the heel of the front foot is as far forward as the tip of the toes of the rear foot). If we're doing low Tai Chi, we separate the feet somewhat more, but not enough to render us immobile; the farther we separate the feet, the more difficult it becomes to move either foot. There's a golden mean there somewhere.

Ultimately it's about being wide enough and long enough to take a shove or a yank from any direction, while also being capable of moving.

Great. So now we take a step, and everything's totally messed up. We're on a tightrope, or we're twisted up, or our feet are pointing in opposite directions. What went wrong?

What went wrong was where and how we set down our stepping foot. Set it down in the wrong place and we're a mess. So we drill. We practice stepping in every direction, and when we err we adjust. We drill stepping daily, preferably without dropping the gaze, until we can reliably come down in a proper stance in any direction.

As we'll see in later chapters, there are other important elements of stance. For now we just want to be wide and long and rooted to the surface beneath us.

Rootedness is more than just setting the feet, of course. It's also where we're putting our energy. In Tai Chi we're connecting our energy to the energy of the earth, which brings us to the second part of this foundational principle.

How do we go about rooting ourselves energetically? The short answer is visualization. Many practitioners visualize a cord of white light being exhaled from the base chakra into the earth. Some see a lightning bolt or a chain and anchor. You can see your body at the center of the earth. Whatever speaks to you, but do try to catch a glimpse of something. Remember that Tai Chi master who couldn't be moved off his spot? Just before the demonstration began, he went off by himself and used visualization to sink his root. That's how it's done.

If you consider yourself a failure at visualization, welcome to the world's largest club. The best advice? Keep it simple. The most important thing is to be clear about what you want to accomplish. That's half of it, if not more. The rest is confidence. Keep a light touch and rest assured that something's happening, whether you're seeing it clearly or not.

20. THE OTHER

In Tai Chi, there's always an
adversary whose presence helps us focus.

We're never alone, you and I. Whether or not our dance partner is visible, we're always in relationship, every moment of our lives. Remember: our art was named after the circle of two fishes, only one of which can be seen. So even when there's nothing there, *nothing* is there. Nothing turns out to be very important in our little enterprise. So we're back to the two fishes, back to solid and empty and how the two relate.

I think it's helpful to see Tai Chi as sacred encounter. It's relationship work, especially if we're practicing Pushing Hands. Even in solo work, we've always got the Other. It can be our adversary, or it can be our beloved, or it can be a helpful fellow student. He or she can have a different identity each moment. To me, it's just the world. Any direction we turn, the world is always there waiting. That's what the Other means to me. The world is a constant presence, and the less we account for that presence, and the less we practice how best to meet the world with poise, and alertness and heart—the less agreeable our lives are going to be.

Carlos Castaneda's books talk about the importance of "a worthy opponent." Otherwise we can get away with sloppiness, and our powers are never fully brought to bear. That's why in Tai Chi we always have a practice partner. It's built in because every Tai Chi posture is designed to face an attacker from a certain direction. That's the nature of the art. In Tai Chi we're constantly resetting ourselves for an attack that could come at any moment or never come at all. We're alert enough for the former and relaxed enough for the latter. Should the world decide to give us a little shove today, we're fully prepared to hold our spot on the planet's surface.

And it *is* our spot. You and I may not be entitled to a lot, but we do hold a land grant to the small piece of earth beneath our feet and the air entering our nostrils, and this should be our abiding attitude.

In Tai Chi, we bring all our attention to the very important business of taking a stand. Of taking a step. Of turning in a new direction. Of backing out of an untenable situation. Of encountering a bully. These are necessary life skills, and our Tai Chi gives us a chance to hone them until we can accomplish them in the real world with confidence and sensitivity and even élan.

How does one go about taking a stand in life? Ask a Cheyenne. Maybe you've heard of the Dog Soldiers, a warrior society among the Cheyenne tribe. A Dog Soldier rode into battle with a leather strap attached to his body. At the end of the strap was a sharpened stake, and what a Dog Soldier did was jump off his horse in the middle of the fray, send the horse packing, sink his stake into the ground and draw his weapon. On that spot, the Dog Soldier fought until he was killed or until one of his brothers came and pulled up his stake.

What I'd like you to do right now is imagine the stance that warrior took when he drew his weapon and took his stand. It was his whole life summed up in a single moment.

That's the place.

Every time we take a stand in Tai Chi, we are the Dog Soldier. The difference is, we're not shot full of adrenaline because we're taking our stand all day long as a matter of course. We're keeping ourselves loose and balanced because ours is a marathon event, but we have no less commitment, okay?

We're every bit as all-in as that young Cheyenne with his stake in the ground, and our stance shows it. No aggression, no paranoia. Just dead-on center.

21. Front Foot Straight, Rear Foot Out

The front foot points straight ahead in Tai Chi,
while the rear foot turns out at a comfortable angle.

In Tai Chi, the front foot always points toward the adversary, whether real or imagined, while the other foot is set to the rear and turned out at a forty-five-degree angle. That's a hard-and-fast rule. Whether our bodyweight is assigned to the forward leg or the rear, we maintain this exact alignment of the feet.

Why? I had a feeling you'd ask. First and foremost, we're protecting the forward knee. When we point a well-bent knee at the Other, he's all but incapable of attacking it. The front of a bent knee is formidable. What we never want to offer the Other is a free broadside.

Why turn the rear foot out at an angle? Because that's how we generate push. If we need to push a car, we turn the rear foot out. Nothing else works. Same thing when it comes to holding our ground. If a sudden shove should come our way, we want to have a push-foot behind us and that foot needs to be turned out. So we're relaxed, we're on center, our knees are bent, our front foot is pointing straight at the Other, and our rear foot is turned comfortably out.

It's how we meet the world.

We're changing the way we hold ourselves. It's subtle, but it's there. You and I will never again float around in a bubble of self-absorption, oblivious to what's around us. We're eyes out, energy out now. We're feeling everybody.

22. KNEE BEHIND TOES

*The knee of a weighted leg
must never extend beyond the toes.*

Here's another principle whose whole purpose is that of protecting the knee. Not from the adversary but from ourselves. In Tai Chi, the knee of a weighted leg must never extend forward of the toes because that really stresses the knee. It's out over empty space.

Imagine holding a bowling ball at arm's length. That's a lot of weight to put out over empty space, right? Even if we used both arms, it would still stress the whole body. Well, you and I weigh a lot more than a bowling ball. Let's not put all that weight bearing down on an unsupported knee. When we place the whole bodyweight out beyond the knee, maybe we get away with it for a few months or a few years, but sooner or later there's going to be trouble.

I went through one aggressive period early in my practice when I was working relatively low to the ground, and finally my right knee got really inflamed. It wasn't until I videoed myself that I understood why. In one particular posture, my weighted right knee was projecting about four inches beyond the toes. I made the correction right away, but it was six months before the pain subsided.

Do this. Stand with one foot set forward of the other. Place most of your weight on that forward foot. Now look down. If you see the tips of your toes protruding beyond your knee, that's exactly what you want. If not, something needs adjusting.

You can adjust your stance by pulling the hips back a little. Or you can raise your hips a little. Or you can adjust the distance between your feet. Play with these variables until you've found something solid and comfortable that protects that forward knee.

Same deal when the bodyweight is over the rear foot. Be sure to check the position of the rear knee. Don't let it overhang the toes.

23. Foot and Knee Always Agree

In Tai Chi, foot and knee
always point in the same direction.

Here's another hard and fast rule that follows close behind the previous two. In Tai Chi, the foot and the knee always point in the same direction. This supports and protects both knee and ankle because they're both designed to be straight-on.

Tai Chi is about using the body according to its design, and the ankle and knee were designed to work together, neither of them twisted out to the side. Foot and knee always agree.

Of course we're always twisting the spine in Tai Chi (see Chapter Forty-Three) and at times there's a temptation to torque the knee *just* a little to relieve pressure on the spine. It's cheating, basically. You're getting a nice big twist just using a modest bit of spinal flexibility by letting the knees and even the ankles twist right along with the upper body. Shame on you. I can assure you I've never done such a thing.

If you don't know what I'm talking about, stand up and twist your upper body as though you're trying to see someone standing behind you—only don't let your knees or ankles twist in the slightest. You feel that strain along your spine and neck? Now do it again, only cheating, letting your lower body twist right along with your spine.

Different? I'll say they're different.

We don't give in to temptation, you and I, because the spine is designed to twist and the knees and ankles aren't. Write it down. Foot and knee always agree.

24. Dripping Foot

A raised foot hangs limp and vertical
in Tai Chi, the toes dripping down.

We're always balanced on one leg in Tai Chi, so we've always got one foot in the air. This principle talks about that raised foot. What we want to do is hold it reasonably close to the ground, hanging vertically with the toes pointing to the earth. This grounds the raised leg visually and energetically and minimizes teetering.

Ankle flexibility allowing, we'd really like to create a perfect vertical line from the knee to the toes. Good luck with that. A nice vertical line in the lower leg parallels the vertical line of the torso and head and unifies the posture. But no cheating; no using muscular tension to straighten the foot—well, maybe just for a second. We want our Tai Chi to be as relaxed as possible, so we're holding that raised foot completely limp, just hanging by the tendons, the toes "dripping" down.

Another thing about the raised foot. When we lift it off the ground, it comes up a bit at a time. We're "peeling" it off the ground, the heel first, followed by the midsole and then the toes. Likewise, when the foot returns to the ground, it returns a bit at a time. If we're setting it down to the side or to the rear, the toes touch down first, followed by the midsole and then the heel.

It's a little different when we set the foot down toward the front. We're peeling it up the same way, we're dripping it down the same way, but the foot flips just before it re-encounters the earth, exposing the heel. It's the heel that makes first contact, followed by the midsole and the toes. We want to accomplish that flip at the very last moment. We maintain the dripping foot as long as we can because it makes for better composition.

A lifted horizontal foot is not only bad design but an actual hazard, hooking table legs and small children. We want that foot pointed down. Think about the basic character of the foot. It's proud but very modest. The foot accomplishes its great work with understatement and dignity, and that's how it expresses in posture and movement. Doing much while being unnoticed.

Finally, a reminder. As we saw in Chapter Fifteen, each of our movements in Tai Chi should describe an arc, and that's certainly true of our dripping foot. As it lifts itself, moves itself and sets back down, the foot should describe an arc, an *El Arco de Triunfo* if you'd like. To learn the language of Tai Chi, to participate truthfully in its art, is a triumph of the soul.

25. EMPTY FOOT, MOVE FOOT, FILL FOOT

To step in Tai Chi, we empty the foot,
then move the foot, then weight the foot.

This principle seems pretty straightforward, but it's the opposite of how you and I normally walk. What we usually do is commit our bodyweight forward then hurriedly begin moving the feet. With luck, we don't trip over anything, and we end up at point B.

It's a little different in Tai Chi.

In our movement art, we don't commit the bodyweight forward until after we have completed the step. We separate those two things entirely. You're stepping then you're shifting. That way, we're never at risk of slipping or tripping, and we're far less vulnerable to leg sweeps (that's where the adversary uses his forward foot to sweep your forward foot from under you—nasty stuff).

Every time we take a step in Tai Chi, we begin by emptying the stepping foot of every trace of bodyweight. *Every* trace. Now we relocate that foot, and it settles unhurriedly against the earth, still completely weightless. Finally, taking our time, we return the bodyweight to the foot.

That process is the same every time. No matter which way we're stepping, we use the same threefold process. Empty, move, fill. Eventually it's seamless, but in the beginning either we're really concentrating on articulating each phase or we're doing it wrong. We have to drill and drill, exaggerating each part of the process until it's automatic.

Everybody cheats. The best way to catch yourself cheating is to freeze just after you've set the stepping foot down. Now lift that foot into the air. Can't? You're busted. You began shifting your weight onto the foot while it was still in motion.

Be serious about doing this right. This principle is about keeping ourselves upright and under control in the middle of chaos. Whether that's crossing an icy parking lot, or negotiating a slippery supermarket floor, or negotiating your way through a riot—whatever it is. Maybe it's about keeping yourself safe with pets and toddlers darting about your feet. We're learning not to commit ourselves forward until we're sure of our footing. Once that becomes our way of moving through life, it doesn't look halting or afraid. It looks present and under control.

I once referred to this principle as Stepping onto Frozen Lake. We want to test the ice with our forward foot before committing our weight. If we hear a cracking sound, we can catch ourselves and withdraw.

The Chinese say we should walk as though stepping on cats. That means soft landings. With this principle we're becoming mindful of how we're meeting the earth. As adolescents, we probably crashed about more or less thoughtlessly. We're past that now. No more needless shocks to the body, nor to that of the living earth. We're growing a little sensitivity. We're growing a little respect.

One cool thing about this principle is something athletes call *hang time*. That's the lon-nnng moment when something—a tossed ball or a leaping body—seems to hang weightless before it begins to descend. It's that magical, timeless interval between going up and coming down that logically shouldn't have duration yet does.

We go there each time we take a step in Tai Chi.

Because we haven't hurried our weight forward, that stepping foot can hang suspended for a very long time as it traces each tiny interval of its lazy arc up then down through quantum space. At the same time, we can raise the hips slightly as the foot rises then lower the hips as the foot falls. The whole body is getting to experience the joy-ride, that achingly magical moment at the top of the arc when everything hangs suspended.

Finally, the whole body settles back to earth like a blanket tossed over a sleeping child. We *drift* back in for a feather-soft landing. It's a little like flying. It really is. Even though we're flying with one foot firmly on the ground.

The first time I saw Tai Chi performed in front of me, my friend Cangming was demonstrating the Twenty-Four in the sand of a playground. What I was doing was checking to see whether his feet were touching the ground. They were, and they weren't. One foot was firmly grounding Cangming's body, yes, but all the rest of him was flying. There were no flat places in his arcs, no nasty collisions with the planet, nor even the merest thought of gravity. It looked for all the world like my friend was doing his Tai Chi just above the ground.

26. FEET COME TOGETHER

*In Tai Chi, the stepping foot first
circles in toward the other foot then circles out.*

Yes, we are still talking about the feet. This principal is one of nine that describes the proper functioning of the foot in Tai Chi. Here we encounter the *crescent step*, as I call it. Every time we take a step in Tai Chi, the feet come together for a moment then separate. This is not emphasized but done in a single smooth motion.

Here's the boilerplate:

Once we've lifted the stepping foot, it circles in toward the stationary foot then circles back out and sets down. The overall effect is that of an arc or expanding spiral. Note that the feet don't actually touch one another. We don't want to trip ourselves up; the whole point is to avoid tripping.

Imagine yourself at a crowded party. You want to cross the room to say hi to someone, so you're picking your way carefully, shuffling along with your feet close together. Otherwise, you're hooking chair legs or people's ankles. That's the whole idea of the crescent step, keeping your base small when in transition.

One important note. As we're making all these lovely arcs and crescents, let's be certain that the knee continues to point forward.

We're circling the foot, not the knee. Practice holding the knee aloft and stationary while the foot circles. It's as though the lower leg is stirring a pot.

There's a practical application here, beyond navigating crowded parties. At times we may need to step forward in a very dark place. Let's say there's a power outage. How best to grope our way to the flashlight? Well, first we want to give our eyes a minute to adjust to the darkness. Then we begin crescent-stepping our way forward, remembering to not commit the weight until the stepping foot has found a safe spot to set down.

More to the point, before it sets down, the stepping foot describes an outward circle, probing the area immediately ahead. We're taking our time and probing. (Meanwhile, our arms and hands are forming a protective circle in front of the upper body; we don't want to blunder into something nose-first.) This is one of many examples of the broad applicability of the principles of Tai Chi.

27. ESTABLISH REAR FOOT FIRST

When we adopt a posture in Tai Chi,
we begin by setting the rear foot in place.

In Tai Chi, we're constantly preparing ourselves to meet the Other in the most appropriate way. Specifically, we want to be facing the Other with a push-foot set firmly behind us.

In any Tai Chi posture, we begin by establishing a push-foot. Then the rest of the body arranges itself around that foot. That's the process. Should the Other jump us before we're fully ready, at least we have that push-foot in place and can remain standing.

Here's an example of what we're talking about. Actually it's a negative example. In the Twenty-Four Movement Form, we're taught to begin by hanging a left and assuming the posture Part Wild Horse's Mane, the *final* detail of which is to establish the push-foot. That's right, we complete the posture and then we set the rear foot.

I'm sorry, but that's a little like drawing the bow, aiming carefully, and then loading the arrow.

If you practice the Twenty-Four, I suggest you experiment with turning the right foot first rather than last. That is, to state it very carefully, after one lifts the arms and bends the knees to begin the sequence, he or she turns the right foot to the left (actually, we're turning the whole body except for the left foot; see Chapter Twenty-Nine), then shifts the bodyweight onto that perfectly positioned right foot for the completion of the move. That way we're on solid ground from the beginning and arrive in the final posture with full authority.

28. Foot Pivots on Heel

*When changing directions
in Tai Chi, we pivot the foot on the heel.*

Whenever we turn the foot in Tai Chi, that foot should pivot on the heel rather than on the ball of the foot. Why? Because once the heel comes up, we've lost our earth connection and can be yanked around quite easily.

Take a good look at the heel. Examine not only the bottom of the heel but the whole structure. It's massive. We can see at a glance that the heel makes for a really good anchor and a really poor sail. Which is to say, it's designed to be down. The heel is designed to push against the earth. It's how we walk, it's how we work, it's how we push a car, and it's how we defend ourselves.

Try pushing a car on tiptoes. Try pushing anything on tiptoes. You can't. Yet many Tai Chi practitioners lift the heel of the rear foot every time they direct energy forward. It drives me crazy to see that. I also see people turning by pivoting on the ball of the foot, with the heel up in the air, and it's the same illogic. It's the antithesis of how Tai Chi works because it's the antithesis of how the body works.

Yes, boxers are always up on the balls of their feet because boxing has rules and a referee, and the opponent isn't allowed to grab you and toss you around. Boxing is about scoring points, which means it's about speed and reach. If you want to win the match, you fight on the balls of your feet. The same applies to the martial arts sparring I've participated in. You're up on the balls of your feet flying around and scoring points.

In the real world?

In the real world, a fight lasts about two seconds. It all comes down to the first punch that lands like it should. If the heels are down when that punch lands, the fight's over.

Why lift the heel, ever? Because we need to reposition the foot. Unless we're kicking or kneeing someone (neither is particularly recommended), there's no other reason to lift the heel. If we're just turning, we can do that by pivoting on the heel itself.

Simple.

In the next chapter, we'll take this idea farther, pivoting the foot from the shoulder. But everything begins with establishing the correct pivot-point. The heel is that pivot-point. It's literally where the rubber meets the road.

29. SHOULDERS TURN FOOT

*The foot never pivots on its own in Tai Chi
but in tandem with the turning of the shoulders.*

In Tai Chi, nothing occurs in isolation. If we're turning one foot, we're turning more than just the foot. If the idea is to face a new direction, why not turn *everything* except the support leg? We can't turn the support leg, the weighted leg, because it's busy anchoring us. But we can pivot the rest of the body in one moment, using the shoulders as a steering wheel.

And the support leg? After accomplishing that grand turn, we can very easily subtract our weight from the support leg and correct it—and we're done. This idea of turning the whole body in unison we call Shoulders Turn Foot because that's the way it looks and feels. The shoulders are our steering wheel.

That's it, basically. We'll close by restating the above as tediously as possible:

When we redirect the body in Tai Chi, we begin by placing all the bodyweight on the rear leg. That leg remains as it is during the turning process. Next we rotate the rest of the body along an axis that runs from the unweighted heel to a point between the shoulders. Once the rotation is complete, the weight is removed from the support leg (still pointing in the original direction) which can now reposition itself, becoming the front leg of the new posture.

Note that whenever we turn in Tai Chi, the direction of turn is always toward the rear foot. That's a given because otherwise we get hopelessly crossed-up. Should we want to turn in the opposite direction, we have to go to a transition stance.

Transitioning in Tai Chi is an art within an art. Strictly speaking, we're always in transition because we never—well, rarely—come to a complete stop in Tai Chi. Once we're grounded in Tai Chi's underlying principles, we can improvise a transition anytime anywhere.

The idea is to do whatever needs to be done without exiting Tai Chi.

30. Control Hip Elevation

*In Tai Chi, we're careful to keep
the elevation of the hips under control.*

We always want a bit of knee-bend in Tai Chi, which is easy enough to control when we're in a stationary pose. When we step, though, the tendency is to become straight-legged then drop back down again. This causes us to bob up and down, which we don't want in our Tai Chi. We want the hips to remain at the same elevation, or at least remain under control. Tai Chi instructors usually state this a little differently, telling students to watch their head height. Your teacher may place a bowl of water on your head to focus you on keeping your head under control.

Actually it has little to do with the head and everything to do with the hips. What we're trying to track is hip elevation, which goes back to the amount of knee-bend we're using. Knee-bend tends to vary when we step because we're distracted by the mechanics of moving, and we're probably also pretty weak in the thighs. So we have to make a focus of keeping our hips under control when stepping in Tai Chi.

Does that mean we never vary hip elevation at all?

There are no nevers in Tai Chi. What's important is to bring everything into conscious awareness. Personally, I like to accentuate an ascending or expanding move such as a kick by swelling a bit, meaning I let the hips rise, and I may accentuate a descending or contracting move by dropping the hips a little. Notice I said *a bit* and *a little*. Jacking the whole upper body up and down is not the idea. The first order of business is to get the knees and hips under control.

31. TUCK THE TAILBONE

In Tai Chi, we curl the
tailbone forward between the legs.

Keep your ass under you. That's a piece of advice from a South Florida Tai Chi teacher whose name I wish I recalled. He's right. We lower our hips in Tai Chi, and we keep them lowered, but that doesn't mean we've got our caboose trailing behind us. The tailbone belongs beneath the torso, and we keep it there by curling it forward between the legs.

In this chapter, we'll see how this principle affects the whole body, but first let's be sure we know what and where the tailbone is, and the sacrum above it. This is important because the spinal column rests on the tailbone and sacrum, and if they're wrong, everything's wrong.

The tailbone is about as long as the ring finger and as wide as your thumb, and it has tiny moving parts. We're not just talking about a vestigial tail here but a vital, active part of the skeletal and energy systems of the body. The tailbone hangs suspended so it floats in space, and it should feel floaty. There should be no tension around it.

Just above the tailbone is the sacrum, a highly important triangular structure that acts as the body's U-joint. Everything meets at the sacrum. Unfortunately most of us have a frozen sacrum because we've spent our whole lives in a chair. You and I want a very live sacrum and tailbone, a wiggle in our walk. A sexy walk is our design, and Tai Chi is about re-entering our design.

When we first wake up the sacrum and tailbone, we may encounter a little soreness, what I call *old tightness*. Our muscles and connective tissues have held tension for so long they've forgotten there's any other way. When that soreness shows up, people may get scared and go back to the sofa.

Listen, when something wakes up, it hurts. It doesn't hurt forever. Stay with it. As long as we're moving naturally and understatedly, it's practically impossible to hurt ourselves. No, I'm not a medical doctor and no, I'm not dispensing medical advice. I'd drop dead first, actually. You and I don't need medical advice. What you and I need is fifteen minutes a day of checking in with our bodies and getting real with what we encounter there. If we're encountering soreness, fine, let's *move* the soreness away.

Once the sacrum and tailbone are loose and moving, the lumbar softens too, and the whole posture is able to reconfigure itself. The tailbone no longer sticks out but curls forward, which takes the curve out of the spine at the waist, giving us a single, gentle arc all along the rear of the body. It makes us far more vertical, which is hugely important in Tai Chi because of rotation, which is crucial to Tai Chi as a martial art.

You can't rotate something that isn't vertical. Ever watch an ice skater spin really fast? They're able to do that because they pull everything in until they're perfectly vertical. If so much as a hand were to stick out, the skater's body would fly out of control. In Tai Chi, we too are very concerned about centering and rotating along a vertical axis, and we just can't do that with our ass sticking out.

We can't do much of anything in that posture. Why do we adopt it? Because our lower backs are so compromised. When we lift a heavy object, we tend to bend forward with our rear sticking out, which sets our postural muscles at a ninety-degree angle to their intended use. Not a good idea.

If we can stay vertical, our rear beneath us, we can lift the world. We really can because we're not using the postural muscles but the massive muscles of the thighs. But that means totally changing the way we use the body. It means first of all getting out of the chair. It means developing a soft vertical posture. It means really strengthening our trunk and legs. It means awakening our sleeping parts and gradually toning them until they're ready to re-enter their design.

It means Tai Chi.

Can't we pretend this troublesome principle doesn't exist? Can't we just do our Tai Chi as stiff as boards in our middle parts? Yes, we can. I say that because that's what the majority of the world's Tai Chi practitioners do. Most of us couldn't find our sacrum and tailbone with a map and a flashlight, and we're doing perfectly fine, aren't we?

Yes, but there's a difference between "doing perfectly fine" and self-transforming. People who don't really loosen and re-configure their posture don't self-transform—and I'm not being critical here. This principle is really hard to absorb and assimilate, and then it's hard to remember.

Happily, though, many Tai Chi practitioners become really adept at tucking the tailbone. Sometimes at a demonstration you'll see a master drop down into what I call *the invisible chair*. He or she lowers the hips until the thighs are parallel to the ground (try it!) and then remains there for a minute or so as though seated upon the air. What's the trick? The trick is developing enough strength and flexibility in the trunk of the body to keep that ass under you. Otherwise you fall backward every time.

If you practice the invisible chair, do so with toes touching a wall. That way your knees can't extend beyond your toes (see Chapter Twenty-Two). Instructor Luke Chan calls this exercise *wall squatting*. It's quite a challenge to see how far you can lower your hips without falling backward. You'll discover it isn't very far.

32. THE EMPTY BOWL

In Tai Chi, the body assumes the shape of
an empty bowl, concave in front, convex in back.

We learned in the previous chapter that the tailbone should be curled forward in Tai Chi, which takes the curve out of the spine at the waist, giving us a single, gentle arc along the rear of the body. The current principle says we want to create that same effect laterally. We want the whole body—except for the neck and head—to curl slightly forward, assuming the shape of an empty bowl.

What does it come down to? Once the tailbone is properly tucked, it's just about separating the shoulder blades a little, letting the shoulders tip slightly forward. This gives the whole body a rounded aspect. If we also spread our elbows and let them float forward just a little, and if we lower our hips enough for the thighs to project forward—now the whole body really does describe an empty bowl, the back rounded and the front concave. We go for this effect in Tai Chi because it's an extension of the body's design; we couldn't force the body to be concave toward the rear if we tried. Thus it's part of the Tai Chi aesthetic.

Do *not* let your head curl forward. We always, always want a tall, vertical presentation of the neck and head in Tai Chi. And we don't want to overdo the shoulder blades part. We're mostly just relaxing the shoulder blades and letting them float apart more or less naturally. At first we may have to exaggerate all this in order to find it, but the end result should be subtle.

Interestingly, when we become the Empty Bowl, the whole of our physicality is embracing its corresponding emptiness. That's rather large, and I hope you can see that it's large. When solid and empty are fully present, neither dominating the other, one actually embracing the other, we become *tai chi*, the grand ultimate. When solid and empty are exactly there for each other, each ending where the other begins, each providing perfect support for the other by being ever more perfectly what the other is not—we become the one-plus-one that equals eleven.

33. HAND AT HIP, HAND AT SHOULDER

Whether raised or lowered, the hand remains in proper relation to the torso.

Tai Chi is about relationship. Visually and energetically, the various parts of the body stay in close relation, and a prime example is the hand and the hip. When the hand is lowered, it comes to rest beside the hip because there's a natural kinship there. Likewise, when the hand is raised, it anchors at the shoulder. We don't want fly-away hands in Tai Chi, so whether the hand is raised or lowered, we keep it close. Not touching but close, with a little space beneath the armpits. The thumb usually points toward the body, which further solidifies the sense of connection.

I was taught to always place the resting hand exactly one hand-width (the width of the hand including the thumb) from the hip. I've since increased that to two hand-widths, and I'll tell you why. One width felt wrong. My armpit was practically closed, and my posture as a whole felt constricted. I like my Tai Chi to be a bit more fluffed-out and expressive. That's me. I'm not saying that has to be you.

I was also taught to park the resting hand exactly opposite the point of the hip, and here too I'm slightly seditious. I prefer to place my hand a full hand-width forward of that point, which enhances the Empty Bowl effect and also creates a nice parallel between the forearm and the thigh.

Further: I was taught to hold the palm of the resting hand absolutely level. Personally, I don't find that position very restful. At the other extreme is the Chen Man Ching variation, Beautiful Lady's Wrist, or Fair Lady's Hand. Chen taught his students to hold the resting hand completely limp. The advantage of the Chen variation is that you have a completely relaxed lower arm and hand, which maximizes chi flow. The aesthetics of Beautiful Lady's Wrist are very nice, too, as the lower arm describes a continuous gentle arc from elbow to fingertip, which parallels the Dripping Foot we learned about in Chapter Twenty-Four.

I split the difference. I let the hand angle down slightly like a roofing tile, which is another common teaching.

But what's the *correct* way to hold the resting hand, you want to know? I'm sorry but the more instructors you work under, the more variations you're going to come across. There's no right way. There's no original way. It ain't out there. Eventually you're just grateful for the whole range of options. It comes down to which variation is right for you. So, what's your personal practice telling you? Everything finally comes down to your own personal practice.

Having said all that about hand position, let's remember that the body is in constant motion in Tai Chi. We aren't just parking the hand somewhere. We're talking about stations that the hand passes through.

When my hand descends to rest position, it never comes to a complete stop but only slows down and slows some more, and then the shoulder does something and the hand whips around *just* before coming to a stop, and we're on to something else. At one moment the hand may be parallel to the ground, at another it's diagonal, and at another it's hanging limp. But there's always a closeness, a connection, between the hand and the hip. That's the point here.

When the hand is raised, it's the same drill only we're talking about the shoulder rather than the hip. In some postures the raised hand projects forward, in others it's closer to the chest or to the ear—but in each case the hand remains in relation to the shoulder; it never drifts too far away. If we maintain some bend in the elbow and the elbow is pointing down, we're keeping the arm grounded to the body and the whole posture grounded to the earth.

34. Hands Below Eyes

The hands never
obstruct the vision in Tai Chi.

In Tai Chi, the hands remain below the level of the eyes. Some traditional postures station one of the hands higher than that, but in general the hands remain below eye level. There are two reasons for that.

First, we don't want to block our vision. Second, as established earlier, the elbow should always be oriented down in Tai Chi, and it becomes difficult to do that once the hand rises above eye level.

So when a posture calls for a raised hand, we just minimize that part of it. If we're doing White Crane Spreads Wings, the hand is held to the side where it doesn't obstruct the vision much, and it's only up there for a moment. If it's Fair Lady Works at Shuttles, we raise the hand above eye level, and again we're mostly okay. But those are the exceptions. The rule is to keep our hands below eye level, and that's what we do.

35. LEVEL SHOULDERS

The shoulders are level and equal
in Tai Chi, each reflecting the other.

This point may seem obvious, but many of us have uneven shoulders and don't know it. Most of us have a strong shoulder and a weak one, and many people unconsciously hold one whole side of the body protectively without realizing it. Here we're devoting a whole chapter to the shoulders because they're so important and so magnetic to free-floating emotional debris. The shoulders hold anxiety and exhaustion and shame. It may be true to say that we are most naked in our shoulders.

For example, people who live in war zones tend to curl their shoulders in and forward. That can become a permanent hunch. People with self-esteem issues? They have the same posture; it's about wanting to become smaller, wanting to disappear.

If that's you, forget the Empty Bowl (Chapter Thirty-Two). For you, it's about learning to lead with your chest. For you, every Tai Chi move should begin with lifting the sternum. The collarbones, meanwhile, are flowing out to the sides, the shoulder blades are flowing down in back, and the chest is expanding with each breath. That's really important for you.

Another common tendency is to "protect" an old injury by holding one or both shoulders a certain way. The actual injury may have healed long ago, but we're still in protection mode.

It's easy to see someone else's postural problems, but it can be devilishly difficult to see our own. What I did one day was take a marker and draw a grid on a mirror. I used a level and straight-edge because this has to be done exactly right. I examined my posture carefully, which meant closing one eye and adjusting my feet so that my nose appeared on the vertical centerline. Then I checked to see if my navel was also on that centerline. Next I checked whether my hips were at the same height. Finally I compared my shoulders, not only seeing where they hit the grid but also whether the two sides matched.

What we're learning is that it's important to have equal left- and right-side development in every part of the body.

As mentioned, a low shoulder may go back to a low hip, and if that's you, don't be too quick to install a shoe insert. That kind of external remedy just sends another wave of adjustments through the whole body, further complicating an already messy situation. Better would be to release and expand the compressed joint, whatever it is (it's most likely the hip).

A good time to track the position of our shoulders is when we raise an arm in Tai Chi. Beginners raise the arm *and* the shoulder, as though reaching for something on a high shelf. No. The shoulder remains in place in Tai Chi. It's the elbow that rises and falls. The shoulder remains in place. Mark also, when directing a push forward in Tai Chi, the shoulder stays where it is. Same thing when we pull the hand back. Stable, level shoulders.

You and I tend to be the last ones to know what's going on in our own bodies, and our Tai Chi practice is about fixing that. First we establish awareness and control—and softness is always a part of that—and then we can play with expression.

36. Tongue at Roof of Mouth

*In Tai Chi, we rest the tip of
the tongue against the roof of the mouth.*

The front part of the tongue is always touching the roof of the mouth in Tai Chi. We're told this completes an important chi circuit. Not that I've personally noticed a lot of difference, but I've heard the same instruction in Zen and yoga and Qigong and Tantra, so by now it's become habit. Every time I think to check my tongue, it's up there. I've come to see it as the natural position of the tongue.

Specifically, we want the tip of the tongue touching the upper palette just behind the teeth. There's a spot there called the alveolar ridge, a very ticklish ridge hanging down from the roof of the mouth. Place the tip of the tongue there, or the tip can touch the teeth with the whole tongue resting against the roof of the mouth. The lips, meanwhile, are lightly touching and the jaw is relaxed.

37. LEFT SIDE, RIGHT SIDE

The ideal is to perform each Tai Chi
posture identically on either side of the body.

In art class, we're told that a symmetrical design is a boring design because it's static. We need to throw things off a bit while still hanging onto balance. It's called *composition*, of which the postures of Tai Chi are great examples. Tai Chi doesn't have a single symmetrical posture. There's no need for one because the body is symmetrical to begin with.

In our movement art, we're taking a symmetrical body and throwing things off a bit. We're giving left and right different things to do while maintaining overall balance. From time to time, we're also flipping assignments left and right, requiring each of our halves to perform identically. This balances the left and right sides of our nature.

Most of us are lopsided. "I'm really right-brained," we may say or, "I'm totally left-brained," as though there's nothing we can do about it. Tai Chi is what we can do about it. We practice every posture identically on either side of the body, and we use a mirror to check ourselves—not just the final position of the posture, but also how we came to be there. We should be looking at the same process, the same grace, power, and coordination on either side of the body.

That doesn't happen overnight. It does happen, though, and it's important that it happens. What we're doing is training our recessive side to step forward occasionally and lead, while the dominant side learns to step back and follow. This can have extraordinary benefits.

So, if the routine we're practicing doesn't present Single Whip, et al, on the left side, we take a little initiative. We teach ourselves the other version, and we drill until we're looking at exactly the same thing left and right.

Further, we might decide to go easy on sports and activities that work only the dominant side of the body. I'm talking about tennis and golf and baseball and softball—pretty much everything with a ball. But if you want to play one of these sports, great. Become ambidextrous. I practice archery, and each day I shoot equally from either side of the body. It's important.

What we're working toward is perfect balance, perfect cross-development. Will we ever attain it? Probably not, but we need to work toward that end until we've at least achieved what artists call *control of the medium*. Until an artist is capable of preparing the paints and controlling the brush, the best he or she can hope for is the fortunate accident. In Tai Chi, our medium is the body, and we need to be capable of achieving a given effect every time we reach for it, on either side, or we're just fooling around.

A lopsided butterfly doesn't migrate to Mexico. It just goes around in circles.

38. THE NINE DIRECTIONS

*In Tai Chi, we orient ourselves by means
of eight lateral directions and a mysterious ninth.*

If you've been practicing Tai Chi for a while, you've noticed that we always orient the body toward one of eight directions. The most common are the four cardinal directions. Sometimes a posture faces into a corner, but it faces *exactly* into that corner. No odd angles. Thus, Tai Chi can be said to concern itself with precisely eight lateral directions spaced forty-five degrees apart. If you're off a little, you're off a mile.

It goes farther. In every traditional Tai Chi posture, each *part* of the body points toward one of those same eight directions. Each knee, the hips, the shoulders, the head, everything orients to one of those eight lateral directions.

The reasoning goes back to *Feng Shui*. Like many cultures, the Chinese have a rich tradition concerning the attributes of the various directions. If your instructor tells you to always begin practice facing the east, or to sleep with your head to the north, it's the same principles at work.

Your instructor may place little or no emphasis on the directions. No worries. We're constantly wheeling about in Tai Chi, so who cares which direction we faced in the beginning? What's important is that we establish one direction as our "true north," and it doesn't have to correspond to the compass. Usually we just begin facing a wall. Fine, as long as we remember the direction where we began. We want to finish facing that same direction.

If the meanings of the directions interest you, read up on them and include them however you'd like. You'll encounter four-directional systems and six-directional systems and seven-directional systems, and so on. Reality can be sliced up as many ways as you wish. It's the relationship among the slices that matters. In Tai Chi we orient ourselves according to precisely eight lateral directions because that's how Tai Chi is built.

And then there's the mysterious ninth direction.

What can really be said of the directionless direction? The Chinese speak of Wu Chi, the primordial emptiness that underlies form, and that's about as close as we can come because we're talking about something that can't be talked about. But neither can it be left out of the conversation.

I'm sure you've heard of *dark matter* and *dark energy*. Those, too, are ways of talking about something that can't be talked about—nor can they be left out of the conversation because they comprise about ninety-five percent of all that is. Chew on that for a moment. Only five percent of existence can be detected by any scientific means. The other ninety-five is what you and I call the black fish, or Wu Chi, or the directionless direction, the center from which every direction issues. In Tai Chi that point is seen as lying at our own center.

I begin and end every Tai Chi sequence with a brief standing meditation, Stand Like a Tree, which has my arms forming a circle in front of my chest. I'm literally holding open a space for my "other" ninety-six percent. I also invoke Wu Chi as part of the Nine Directions Form, an original sequence I composed in 2004. We each need a way to touch the sacred mystery at our center, and our daily movement practice provides the perfect opportunity.

I encourage you to compose your own Tai Chi sequences, as I do. See the various postures of Tai Chi as vocabulary elements to combine in endless variations. As long as we begin and end our sequence standing in the same spot, facing the original direction, we're well within tradition.

PART THREE: COMING TO LIFE

In Part Two, we examined a double handful of technical principles that orient us in spatial and gravitational reality. We learned that a Tai Chi practice must be built from the ground up. If you're now doing that foundational work, if you're becoming technically sound in all those details—great. That puts you in a very select group of practitioners.

And yet.

If we never go beyond "technically sound," we've left a lot of money on the table. In this final section, we go beyond technique into . . .

Well, let's turn the page and see how one even begins to talk about *coming to life* in our personal movement practice.

39. COMMITMENT

In Tai Chi, we totally commit to whatever
we're doing, feeling, and expressing this moment.

"He commits."

That's a strong compliment for an actor. Maybe a scene calls for something as simple as lifting a coffee cup and taking a small sip. Even that requires commitment. It requires making that cup your own. It requires noticing the exact taste and temperature of the coffee, even if the cup is in fact empty. Maybe a scene calls for an act of cruelty or hatred. You have to go there. You have to find those places within yourself and commit to them.

It's the same in Tai Chi. When a certain move appears in a Tai Chi sequence, we must find where it lives in ourselves and go there. Just as in theater, our response may be very different on different days. Today Slant Flying may bring up a mysterious stab of anger. Tomorrow the same move may summon a sense of longing. What's important is that we're *here*, present with what's being called for, and with what's welling up in us, both. We are where the two meet.

A Tai Chi move can be thought out in advance and practiced hundreds of times, but a moment can't be planned because it doesn't belong to us. We can't know its nature even an instant before.

We're not thinking or forcing our way forward, you and I. Not anymore. We're feeling our way forward, and what comes up, comes up. Our job is to notice that unexpected something, to receive the unannounced visitor, to *become* that visitor and never look back. That should be our every moment in Tai Chi.

Something else actors like to talk about is *high stakes*. A scene must have high stakes, it's said, or there's no reason for the actors or the audience to care. Same in Tai Chi. We're making life-or-death decisions each instant. What are we doing this moment? Lifting one foot and turning? That's all, yet our immortal soul hangs in the balance. That has to be our attitude.

Once we've completed our turn, do we linger with it, giving it an extra little flourish—or do we quickly cut to the next move? Every second brings another complex of life-defining decisions. In Tai Chi, each decision we make carries the same importance. Each sums up everything we've ever believed, cherished, or wished for.

Remember the Dog Soldier in Chapter Twenty? He staked himself to one spot on the battlefield and fought to the death on that spot. Why that particular spot, we might ask? What was so wrong with that pleasant level spot over there? Or the one with the nice mound of clover? Surely such an important decision deserves a bit of thought, no?

No. It's the commitment itself that fetches the magic. Not what's being committed to.

Here's what happens in Tai Chi. When you or I start into a move, something comes up in us. Maybe it's the same thing that came up the last hundred twelve times we did the move. Maybe it's something completely different. Maybe all we feel is our uncertainty; all we're getting right now is that we don't *know* what we're getting right now. Fine—we go with that. Our move becomes an honest expression of our uncertainty.

What's interesting is: once truthfully enacted, once fully surrendered to, our uncertainty becomes something else. It is transfigured, and we with it. Everything in sight is suddenly something else, lifted a half-notch by our truthfulness. I don't exaggerate when I say that nothing will ever be the same again, even on the far side of the world. That's why I say Tai Chi is alchemy. That's why I say it's a service we do.

Commit.

In your daily Tai Chi practice, if you're doing nothing more than bow—*bow,* for the love of God. Bow from your bones. Until you have truthfully bowed, the whole universe stands waiting. Give it the time and space it requires. Do. The. Deal. Fall through your inner spaces until you've located the spot from which you bow, and let that place bow for you. Or caricature it. Send it up. I don't care what you do. I care very much how much commitment you give it.

Watch a really good Tai Chi practitioner. He or she may begin moving with a certain attitude, then there's a perplexed pause. It's as though he or she is listening to something no one else can hear. Suddenly everything changes. Then another impulse rises, and with it comes another change in coloration, or mood, or motivation. On and on, arrival after arrival. That's presence. That's commitment. That's the theater of self, which is what Tai Chi is most essentially about.

We are shape-shifters, you and I. We are becoming we know not what. Our business is that of surrendering to the unknown creature only now welling up in us. Maybe the most truthful thing we can say about ourselves is: we are an impulse rising *just* now in universal mind. If we can be transparent to that upwelling, we can be one with the mind in which it occurs.

40. Shared Gestures

*Different parts of the body
often share a gesture in Tai Chi.*

Maybe you've had this experience. You're doing this Tai Chi move or that one, and you realize that your right foot and your left hand are doing the same thing at the same time. They're sharing a gesture. Maybe they're moving at the same speed in the same direction. Then maybe they slow and rotate as one. But there's a pairing. There's a connection. There's a relationship.

That happens all the time in our Tai Chi. Sometimes I use the term *discovered correspondences* or, when I'm feeling poetic, *two flags in the same wind*. Call it what you like. Tai Chi is about relationship.

We really should work on relationship, you and I, because if there's one human failing that can end us between now and the middle of next week—it's relationship. We don't feel our connection to others. We don't feel our connection to the earth. We know we're all one and the Earth is our mother, but it's just words banging around in our heads. You and I are staring extinction in the eyes because we don't *feel* what we know to be true, and Tai Chi is a direct response to that problem.

I say it begins with feeling what's going on in ourselves. How are we supposed to feel the plight of people starving in Africa when we're not even half aware of what's going on inside ourselves?

Take your left ribcage. Really, take that rack of ribs and spend a moment finding out what's going on with it and who its friends are. Right away we're aware of certain things. First of all, we are noticed. When we (the locus of attention) show up in the ribcage for a visit, we can expect surprise followed by a flurry of greetings and a general sharing around of information. All this occurs on the level of feeling, which may or may not include subtle visual or even verbal aspects.

Just to expand on that for a moment, you and I can send our awareness into any part of the body anytime, and it's a pity we aren't taught this at a young age. Instead, when we have symptoms, we're sent to a doctor to learn what's going on inside us. Why? Why not just send our awareness into the heart or the stomach and ask, "How exactly are you? What's the story with these symptoms lately?"

I say we get an answer every time. Maybe (probably) it's not verbal, but why should it be? Why, in fact, are we so oblivious to our heart or our stomach that a question is even required? How can we know the distance from the Earth to the Sun—and not know the condition of our own organs?

It's called failure to feel, and it's why we need Tai Chi.

Anyway, when we're focused on our left ribcage, one of the things we may notice is that it feels a strong affinity with the left elbow. Why would it not? They hang together a lot. They sleep together. There's a shared sense of home and identity and priority, and you don't really know either of them until you're feeling that shared sense.

From my own observations, the elbow sees the ribcage as a port of refuge. That's where it anchors. The ribs, meanwhile, see the elbow is a companion and a protector. Up to a point, the two can be separated without any big problem, but only up to a point. That's because of the fine energetic webbing that connects them.

Imagine a spider's web made from filaments of light. That webbing is very malleable so it can stretch and contract with our movements, but there's a point where it gets stretched a bit too thin. When we lift our elbow really high, we feel the webbing stretch farther and farther until it breaks.

That's not a serious problem because the web reknits the instant the elbow returns, but for that one moment the elbow and the ribcage are out of touch. They literally don't feel one another, and that feels wrong to both parties.

Don't take my word for any of this. Try it. With your awareness in your ribcage, slowly raise your elbow. Do you sense a subtle connection that stretches thinner and thinner until, at a certain point, it snaps? Now bring the two gradually closer. Is there a point where they re-connect? The answers are yes and yes, whether or not you can presently feel it going on. You will.

Why is all this so important to Tai Chi? Because we're constantly arranging the body in various ways, and we need to know immediately when something is out of its proper place. We need to feel the pleasure that comes from a body in proper relation, and we need to feel that *snap* that means we've just broken a connection.

When our body parts are feeling each other, and *we're* feeling that feeling being felt—magic happens. The body becomes a language shared with itself. When a hand perfectly mirrors the movement of a foot—magic happens. When a forearm creates an exact parallel with a thigh—something special happens. That's especially true when the conversation involves the two sides of the body because now the two sides of the brain are working in tandem.

Our Tai Chi is showing us that nothing occurs in isolation because nothing can occur in isolation. We're learning to see ourselves as communities of communities, nested one inside the other, each self-aware and relating, each intelligent and creative and yearning to learn and grow and become what it cannot presently imagine.

Importantly, relationship isn't something that has to be invented. We just *notice* that our blood moves from a sense of community. We notice that every time a muscle contracts, a complementary muscle lengthens. We notice that when we're in need of sleep, sleep comes. We notice when one part of our body beckons to another and the other timidly replies.

We see everything as a dance of bashful partners, passionate partners, devouring partners. In Tai Chi, we step into the middle of that dance of co-becoming and we open it out as wide as possible because, at the deepest level, that's what we are. We *are* the principle of relationship.

41. The Golden Thread

Transitions should be seamless in Tai Chi,
each posture flowing naturally into the next.

Beginners in Tai Chi are taught to pause at the end of each move, and the reason is quite simple. The instructor needs a moment to check everyone's form. It's a teaching convention. Tai Chi is not designed for all those stops and starts. You and I are not commuter trains. What we're looking for in Tai Chi is a gradual, natural evolution of events, a continuous flow that keeps the energy moving forward. It's as though a golden thread runs through the whole sequence, connecting each posture, each moment. We don't want that thread to break.

Not to say we never stop stock-still in Tai Chi. Occasionally (see Chapter Forty-Five), we do. Sometimes we slow to the point where we *seem* to arrive at a complete stop, but in nearly every case we're not actually stopping. At that last delicate moment, just as it seems we're stopping stock-still, we find ourselves pulled gently forward by that golden thread.

To say it differently, the seeds of the next move are always stirring to life in the present one. If someone tells you they can't tell where one move ends in your Tai Chi and the next begins, take it as a compliment.

In Tai Chi, every moment is equal. That means our transitions deserve just as much care and development and focus as our end positions.

What is an end position anyway? It's a photo op. Pick up any Tai Chi book and you'll find lots of pictures of people proudly staging their end positions. Happily, Tai Chi is not a photo op but a living, ever-evolving process of *oozing* forward into pure mystery. You can take a photo of a position in Tai Chi. You cannot take a photo of Tai Chi.

42. The Swan

*Tai Chi is beauty
for beauty's sake.*

People come to Tai Chi for all kinds of reasons. Certainly many come to bask in the sheer beauty of the experience. Artists gravitate to Tai Chi because *we* are the work of art we're developing. When we paint, all the beauty goes onto the canvas. When we sculpt, all the beauty winds up in the piece. In Tai Chi we uncover our own native beauty moment by moment. This we do by progressively discovering and falling back on our original design, retracing the original brush-strokes of the creator's hand.

In his book *The Joyous Cosmology*, Alan Watts describes a universal impulse toward beauty. Things flow toward their own perfection, he suggests, because beauty wishes to complete itself. Darwinians try to explain away gorgeous forms and colors by pointing out their practical utility. It's all random mutation and survival, they say. And I reply: why would such a universe want to exist?

I know why a beautiful universe wants to exist.

Said John Keats, "Beauty is truth, truth beauty. That is all ye know on earth and all ye need to know." I agree with Keats and Watts that we need to stop thinking of beauty as the garnish on the side of the plate. We need to stop seeing it as synonymous with *cute* or *pretty*. Sometimes beauty is neither. The larval stage of a butterfly isn't an attractive sight, nor is childbirth. Yet in each case a powerful impulse is at work. Once realized, a living creature's crowning achievement, its perfection, reaches back in time and colors every awkward stage along the way as equally breathtaking.

Maybe the definition of love is being able to see that eventual perfection during each awkward stage along the way, keeping one's sight on the beauty at the core of each of us. That's the traditional Navajo way. When a Navajo looks around and sees an ugly, cynical world, he or she goes to the shaman and says, "My heart isn't right." That person goes in search of healing because an ugly world is a personal failing.

I like that way of seeing it.

You and I can go to a shaman, or we can go to our practice space. There we can experience beauty without end because it emanates from us. It was placed in us at our inception. What we're going for in our practice is eliminating the gap between our original design and what we've come to be. When the two are one—with neither compromised—that's the place.

Why do I refer to this principle as *The Swan?* Because I've seen one. To witness a wild swan emerge from the chill morning mist with another swimming along its side is to absolutely know the universal impulse toward beauty, and to know we can never be separate from it. What other impulse could possibly give rise to such a creature? Or to an orchid? Or to you?

Okay, some details now. If you're trained in the arts, great. That means you understand composition and narrative. Let's talk about composition first, beginning with focal point.

Artists know that every good design has a focal point, meaning one spot the eye is drawn to. In a charcoal drawing, the focal point may be the darkest spot, or in a painting, the boldest splash of color. Sometimes the focal point is defined by two or more converging lines leading the eye to one spot. Other lines, meanwhile, may pull the eye away from the focal point and re-circulate it back through the composition.

Without this kind of attention to narrative and unfoldment, we don't have a design. We have wallpaper. In the same way, each moment in our Tai Chi needs a clear focal point, or our composition is scattered and ineffectual.

Notice how in Tai Chi all the interest is sometimes concentrated in what the right hand is doing. As we watch, we can see that the hand is *leading* the rest of the body into a unified gesture. Then the interest shifts elsewhere, maybe passing from the right arm through the shoulders to the opposite arm, or the two arms may circle down to a rising knee that then becomes a kick. The whole body is participating; everything is in motion, yet at the same time something is leading, pulling everything else along.

It's frequently one of the hands that leads the body, that captures the attention of an observer—but we don't want to become just a pair of hands. Most of us tend to lead with our dominant hand, in particular, and we need to watch that tendency.

What we want is to move the focal point from one body part to another. Good Tai Chi composition circulates the eye throughout the body with circular shapes and motions. We're drawing the eye along an interesting pathway—which brings us to the subject of narrative.

Narrative art is composition that moves forward in time. An obvious example is music, which cannot be experienced in a single moment. Another example is literature; we read one word at a time, and our minds are conducted along a pathway of experience. Literature uses terms like rising action, falling action, climax, and so on. The same elements apply in music and dance and cinema—anything that involves time—and that certainly includes Tai Chi.

Because it unfolds in time, Tai Chi tells a story even when it doesn't intend to. That's just how the mind receives it. The mind is a story-making machine, and when preparing a Tai Chi presentation we're wise to keep that in mind.

Typically that means a gradual build-up of energy culminating in a climactic moment, perhaps a violent strike accompanied by a cry, then the energy winds down and finally we melt back into the spot where we began. Call it the hero's journey. Call it a sexual metaphor. Whatever we choose to call it, it's a story about us. It's the human journey through time condensed into narrative art.

43. TWIST THE SPINE

Every Tai Chi move should
include a full spinal twist and untwist.

Very early on, we established that we want a consistently vertical spine in our Tai Chi. Yet the spine must also be rubbery enough for waves of movement to pass through. Know what else we want? We want a full spinal twist-and-untwist in everything we do in Tai Chi. Every move. Every posture. Every time.

Except for the exceptions.

It may be more accurate to say we want a full twist-untwist as part of our *transition* between Tai Chi postures because it's the twist-untwist that actually takes us from posture to posture. Until we're seeing that and doing that, we're probably waving our arms around a lot. No, no. In Tai Chi, the arms are all but motionless. It's the spinal twist-and-untwist that's animating those arms.

This principle was presented to me as Turn the Waist, which I found exquisitely confusing. I didn't understand how the waist could turn in isolation. I would look down at my waist and say *turn*, and it would just look back at me. My Chinese friend Cangming insisted that the waist did in fact turn, which served to stretch, massage, and tone the organs of the abdomen.

Years later I came to understand that we don't so much turn the waist as twist the spine. This we accomplish by opposing our hips and shoulders. When the shoulders turn and the hips don't, the whole torso, *centered* at the waist, torques and un-torques, and this does indeed stimulate the internal organs and give the many joints of the spine a nice workout. Further, the twist-untwist animates the arms and delivers them to their proper position at the conclusion of the move. So, yes, the waist turns but only in conjunction with the twisting and untwisting of the spine. That's my take.

The process is much like winding up a toy then letting it unwind. As we initiate a Tai Chi move, we give the spine a full ninety-degree twist. That winds up the toy, creating tension and thus potential. As we approach the completion of the move, we release the tension and the toy unwinds, and the body resolves itself in the final position. It's a beautiful, elegant process. It's also a way of delivering considerable power, as we'll see.

First let's look at timing, which is crucial. Every movement has to time out such that the whole body resolves at the same moment. Say our move involves taking a forward step: we want our spinal twist to reach maximum torque at the halfway point of the step. That moment comes just as the stepping foot is passing close to the stationary foot. At that moment, when the feet are close together, the forward shoulder and the forward knee should be *pointing in the same direction*, the direction of the step. That's a really good checkpoint.

Then, as our stepping foot completes its journey, the toy is unwinding, the shoulders are returning to their natural alignment, and everything is falling into place at the same moment.

Timing, they say, is everything. Not only is it tidy and visually pleasing, it's also how we deliver power. When the untwisting of the body coincides with a hand strike—you can see how that adds hot sauce to the strike.

Okay, a detailed example.

When we're doing Brush Knee Push: as the push-hand slowly rises to shoulder level, we're simultaneously twisting the upper body toward the rear leg, in effect winding up the toy. Then, as the stepping foot descends, we begin untwisting, which propels the push-hand gently forward. (Note that the whole body is now behind the push; that's what I mean by delivering power.)

If you're currently a little tight in the joints and can't accomplish a full ninety-degree spinal twist—just do what you can. Leave the shoulders a little short. Do *not* cheat the knee around. That would compromise our stance, and we never want to do that in Tai Chi. Be especially mindful during the Rollback part of Grasp Sparrow's Tail. Do not let that forward knee cheat over to the side.

I know, I know. This principle is hard to get right. But listen, I've seen a lot of Tai Chi practitioners who never twist the spine at all and, God bless them each and every one, those people look like they're from *Night of the Living Dead*.

44. FIRST DO THE OPPOSITE

*A movement in Tai Chi is best initiated
by a feint in the opposite direction.*

Things grow out of their opposites. The lovely lotus, we're told, springs from the murky swamp. Likewise, in Tai Chi we frequently begin a movement with a gesture in the opposite direction. If we're going to turn the shoulders to the right, for example, we may begin by turning them a little to the left. We may even turn them very slightly to the right *before* turning them to the left, before wheeling decisively to the right.

This little feint of ours can be a big production that involves the whole body, or it can be just a momentary waffle of the shoulders. But even that momentary waffle is important, as it sends a relaxing wave through the body that can then resolve itself in the intended movement.

Maybe at times we get a little carried away and our little waffle keeps waffling until it takes over the government. Not a problem. Every movement is equal in Tai Chi, and we can emphasize our wiggle more than the whole succeeding move if we so decide. We need to be open to that kind of impulse. Whatever's coming up, we're making a space for it.

Maybe you've watched a Chen stylist and seen that whole waffling bit. I love Chen stylists because of how loose and expressive they are in their movements. Yang can be a little starchy. In Chen you're always churning, always roiling, always waffling, always feeling your way toward something. Listen, that shouldn't just describe Chen style. That should describe our Tai Chi.

I'll give you an example of what I'm talking about with this principle.

We're approaching a move, let's say one that involves a turn to the right, and we're casting about for the impulse that would lead to that exact movement. So, as we cast about, maybe our shoulders are bobbing left and right, left and right, which helps us generate both the looseness and the impetus to make that right turn. Again, our little prelude may be very brief and understated—then again, we're always coming from a sense of personal discovery in Tai Chi. So we can just *emote* and feel our way forward and let the details sort themselves out.

The last thing we want to be is frozen in place, is the point. We have to generate *some* kind of movement before it can evolve into something else.

Sometimes a waffle can become an explosion. That, too, is more common to Chen style but is the domain of all Tai Chi. What we're doing is tapping into something called *fa jing*. That's a sudden eruption of power that comes from being very, very loose. In karate, they understand that power comes from speed. What they often miss is that speed comes from looseness. That's where our little waffle comes in.

Just before the strike (if the bad guy's willing to wait), we take a moment to shake off our tension and go very transparent. We go so transparent we may not even remember anything about a strike— what strike? Then, when we finally arrive at pure femininity—*boom*! We launch the guy.

Again, things grow out of their opposites.

45. River or Mountain

In Tai Chi, either every part of us
is moving or every part is still.

In Tai Chi, either we're completely in motion or we're completely still. No mix and match. We don't just move the left hand, for example, while the rest of the body is standing there watching.

If the left hand needs moving—fine, let's *all* move the left hand. Every part of us buys in.

We begin by rotating in the opposite direction, shifting the bodyweight toward the rear leg as we withdraw the hand a little. Our gaze is softly focused beyond the open palm. In the space between withdrawing the hand and sending it forward—all eternity holds its breath. In that vast expanse of time, the hand opens slightly, as though in wonder at the enormity of what it's a part of. Finally the spine untwists, the weight shifts in the direction of the hand movement, the breath goes out, and we abandon ourselves to our destiny.

All of that impels that hand on its journey. Either that, or it wasn't worth doing in the first place.

All or nothing. That's the message. If we are the river, every droplet is moving, animating the swirls and eddies, bearing along every twig, everything that's ever happened to us.

You should see me in my kitchen. I'm reaching for the saltshaker and—suddenly I'm the river. I'm balanced on one leg, shoulders bobbing as I gaze fixedly at the saltshaker. Nothing else exists—*only* the plucking of the saltshaker. Depending on the day, there may be considerable vacillating and soul-searching, and the food on the stove may scorch a little—but in the grand scheme of things, who's to say if anything I ever do will matter a whit more than the plucking of the saltshaker?

All moments are equal in Tai Chi.

It's the same with stillness: everything or nothing. When we decide to become still for a moment, we become the mountain. The tides of mind cease. The breath stops. The blood ceases to pulse in our veins. Eternity pauses and waits, spellbound. An ice age passes without comment. Finally, gradually, a thaw begins and we rock gently back into motion. We're once more the river.

So, you ask, when are we supposed to be the river and when the mountain? There's no supposed to. Certainly most of our time in Tai Chi is given to movement; I'd say probably ninety-five percent. You'll find that certain postures call for a moment of stillness; the final position of Golden Rooster Stands on One Leg is a good example. But it can come anywhere. Listen to the moment. Listen to your body. And remember, stillness is not stiffness. We're always soft and listening.

Personally, if I'm moving and my attention begins to wander, I go straight to mountain posture. The sudden shock of stillness brings me back to the moment. After ten or more seconds of stillness, the novelty begins to wear off and I go back to movement, which again refreshes my attention. Again, we're using two extremes to locate ourselves at the center. Sound familiar?

46. THE COLOSSUS

*Tai Chi is about
inhabiting our true immensity.*

This principle means we're large. We're very large. You may have heard of the mythical lumberjack so tall he had to climb a ladder to shave his own face. In Tai Chi, we are that lumberjack. When we lift our hand, we stir the stars. When we shift our weight, we spawn mountain ranges. When we wheel about to face a new direction, we spin off hurricanes.

And we're not just being mythical here. According to the world's great spiritual teachers, if we but glimpsed a fraction of our true enormity, we'd be staggered. You and I *are* the Colossus, one foot in Africa, the other in Europe. We claim this truth for ourselves and for the whole human family each time we practice Tai Chi.

Think of the long, improbable ribbon of family lineage disappearing into past and future—that lineage depends on us. *Everything* depends on us. It's fully on you and me whether mankind discovers the audacity to self-actualize. We must grasp that chance now, in our one fleeting moment of power.

47. Now Yielding, Now Powerful

Tai Chi alternates moments of passivity with moments of explosive power.

Tai Chi is generally seen as a feminine occupation. True, we work on perfecting our passivity in Tai Chi—but that's only half the picture. There are, too, sudden outbursts of power in Tai Chi. Remember fa jing in Chapter Forty-Four? A fa jing strike is as sudden and violent as a lightning strike. So, yes, we're generally very soft and yielding in our art, but we occasionally come from our other side as well.

That bad boy: our masculine side.

The feminine side of Tai Chi is very attractive right now because it's what's missing in our world; thus, a somewhat fey expression of Yang style has become synonymous with emergent Western spirituality. I get it. You and I need to concentrate on opening a space for the feminine right now. But it's not just the feminine that's missing, okay? I don't think we know how to be feminine *or* masculine anymore.

Every day I see good people, and this includes a lot of men, who've no idea how to come from their firmness, who never quite give themselves permission to say *I'm here and I ain't moving.* Occasionally that has to be said. It can be said with humor, it can be said with kindness, it can be said artfully, but it needs to be said.

Women began working on that side of themselves decades ago, and when I look around I see more balanced women than balanced men. The men seem either hopelessly stuck in machismo or running from their masculinity as fast as they can. That's why you see so many men's groups these days. We're confused. We men desperately need to hammer out what it means to be a good, happy man, and until we do that the world will continue to stumble toward oblivion.

I'm really proud of what the feminine sex has accomplished in the past half century. They've stood tall and said, "I don't need a man to provide me with social power or personal meaning. I can find those myself." Very true. And very noble. But allow me to add an additional point. Women have come just about as far as they're capable of coming alone.

In order to take that great final step in their self-realization, women need self-realized men. The kind of radical opening a woman is capable of requires a safe enclosure, a knowing and accepting embrace, or she'll never quite accomplish the beautiful surrender she was designed to invoke for both of them. I'm not talking about sexism here. I'm talking about sexual alchemy, emotional alchemy, relational alchemy; I'm talking about everything set forward as true in Taoism and reflected in the yin-yang circle.

This is our work cosmically, as a society, in our relationships, sexually, personally—and it's certainly our work in Tai Chi. Before the world can find completion, you and I must find completion, and that means developing in ourselves a mature femininity and an equally mature masculinity.

In our daily Tai Chi practice, let's be increasingly aware of our rising and falling tides, our pressing forwards and fallings back, the ever shifting winds of assertion and surrender.

What we're learning is: there is no correct fish. When we choose, we lose. Yet in a practical sense, this principle is saying *let's not forget the masculine side*. We need to whisper that advice to ourselves from time to time because these days masculinity is seen as wrong before it begins, and that's a tragic error. We are both sides of the equation or there's no equation to talk about.

48. Send the Chi

In Tai Chi, we become very
intentional about our use of subtle energy.

Anyone can send energy. We do it all the time. If you've ever prayed for someone, you've sent an organized waveform through the consciousness field, and you can be sure it arrived where and as intended. Even a momentary thought of someone is an organized waveform that's received on some level. The Chinese say *chi follows yi*, meaning energy follows attention.

I learned as a schoolchild never to stare at the back of someone's head in the lunchroom because that person invariably turns to see where the energy is coming from. You can't turn the attention off, and you can't keep it from creating. It's always somewhere doing something, and that can be to our benefit or to our detriment. Random use, random results.

Way back in Part One of this book, we began talking about the inner glow and how to catch sight of it. We practiced moving our locus of perception and becoming intentional about attention. You and I have traveled a great distance since then, and not as tourists but as alchemists in training, and we now have to take responsibility for where our attention is every moment.

Let's practice. Let's get to work gathering and focusing the attention. Let's take a moment now and place our curiosity inside the right forearm. With eyes open or closed, we just let our curiosity dwell there for a few seconds, long enough for a little chi to gather in the lower arm. After a little chi has accumulated there, let's begin unhurriedly moving the attention down the forearm to the wrist. If we focus and take our time, we should be able to feel the chi following quite obediently behind the attention. It's click-and-drag, basically, just a bit slower.

Let's keep it moving, walking our curiosity from the wrist down to the right palm. Once we're feeling some glow in the palm, let's then move our attention from the right hand to the left hand. We're sending our curiosity through the air now, from one hand to the other. Maybe we visualize something passing through the air, maybe we don't. One way or the other, energy will follow the point of attention.

Keeping the experiment going, we can send our attention up through the shoulders, creating a circuit. We're leading our chi in a continuous loop now, through the hands, through the shoulders, and back around. After spending a minute or two cycling the energy this way, reverse the flow for an equal length of time. When we're moving chi, it's generally a good idea to move it equally one way and the other. Another good practice is to finish any kind of energy work by circling the hands over the belly, the dan tien, while intending for chi to be equally distributed and balanced throughout.

Want to take it a little farther? Next time repeat the experiment holding a fresh-plucked leaf between your hands. (Ask permission of the plant first and thank it by presenting some kind of gift.) Feel anything different? Now try sending chi through a sheet of aluminum, a piece of plastic, a word written on a scrap of paper, a crystal. Just play and notice. What happens when you pass chi through the hand of a friend? What impressions do you and your friend receive?

You have to get married now, you know.

What we learn through our experiments in energy work is that, not only can we send chi at will, but also we can also draw energy to us. The better part of most Qigong exercises is pulling chi in from the environment and storing it in our energy system. Many Qigong practitioners make a daily practice of placing their hands on a tree, for example, and drawing chi from it. I've been taught to do the same with distant mountains and even distant planets. There's really no limit. Just remember to say please and thank you.

Seriously, we ask permission before pulling energy out of something. We just step into our humility and put the question out there. If we feel we're receiving an affirmative answer, great, we go ahead. If we're not so sure, we can always pick another tree.

And we give something back in return. A simple thank-you is a good start. Better, we can reverse the flow for a few seconds and send a blessing of good health and long life into the tree, or the distant planet, or whatever it is.

Manners matter. Generosity matters. We have more to give than we know. Our blessings are more powerful than we dream.

One of the really interesting things about energy work is that we can place our attention on something that doesn't yet exist, and energy will gather around that thing exactly as if it presently existed. Chi doesn't know whether something is actualized or not. It just goes where the attention goes. So, by placing our inner sight on an idea, a possibility, a vision of the future, we're surrounding that vision with life-force energy and bringing it closer to realization.

If one of my friends tries to draw me into a discussion about the Illuminati, or secret concentration camps, or massive extermination campaigns—I refuse to participate. If necessary, I leave the table. I know there's plenty of evidence to back up those worst-case scenarios, but, in a universe of infinite alternative realities, why choose that one? Why give my attention to a reality that has all my loved ones behind razor wire, or dead, or crouching in caves? There are other Earths coming into being where human life is stepping into a golden age.

Many trains leaving the station. Which one do you choose to be on?

What our friends, yours and mine, have to learn is they're talking to someone who knows the power of attention and has steadfastly resolved to never use it against his loved ones—which is pretty much everyone here.

Don't call this New Age thinking. It was way back in 1801 that Thomas Young proved that light was neither particle nor wave until touched by consciousness. Once *seen* as particle or wave, light had no choice but to comply. It used the power of human attention to collapse probability array into fact.

That's how things work. Human attention is the hinge upon which destiny swings. At every moment we are Robert Frost's traveler in the yellow wood, pausing at a crossroads. Once a direction has been chosen, all other possibilities close off. You want to close off the possibility of a golden age? It's yours to do. Chi follows yi every time.

I'm not saying we should refuse to carry along an umbrella because that thought may cause it to rain. We're not becoming obsessive or superstitious here. It's completely innocuous to grab an umbrella on the way out the door. I'm saying we don't intentionally focus our attention on (read: blather on about) an outcome we don't want to experience.

Our daily Tai Chi practice is our laboratory of creation. In my movement practice, I don't just perform numbered sequences over and over again. I enact and invoke. My movement sequences are carefully composed and are accompanied by thoughts such as "Beauty before me; beauty behind me; beauty walks beside me; beauty all around me . . ." I open my arms and affirm, "I chose to live heart-first."

These and other movements and meanings have come to me in my personal practice, and I use them very intentionally. It costs no more. It requires no extra time. And listen, we're always creating something. We've no choice in that.

49. AUDACITY

Finally the student must leave behind
every teacher and teaching and go it alone.

You may have heard the story of Zen's Seventeenth Patriarch, a humble temple cook who was asked, "What would you do if you met the Buddha on the road?" His gruff answer was "Kill him and feed his body to the dogs!"

Actually, the Seventeenth Patriarch *became* the Seventeenth Patriarch because of that particular reply, which expressed a very delicate point:

Obedient devotion takes us only so far. There comes a point where we have to forsake our heroes and saviors and teachers and go it completely alone. We take on our own shoulders the cruel yoke of responsibility for what we do and why and how. Otherwise we have failed ourselves *and* our heroes and saviors and teachers.

Killing the Buddha on the road is required. Don't expect it to be enjoyable. There's an actual connection we sever, and it's painful for everyone concerned. That's why the answer to the *koan* is so fierce. We can't just give the Buddha a little slap with our glove. Timidity doesn't cut it here. We have to risk deeply offending everyone we've ever worked with in order to take our first authentic step in Tai Chi. That's why so few people ever take it.

Ultimately the Buddha abandons us, is the thing. Our lineage abandons us. Sooner or later the teachers and the books and the gee-gaws on our altar all walk out on us and we're left with nothing but our bodies and a moment like any other. But if we can muster the audacity to seize that moment and array the universe around ourselves like the creator-gods we are—the result will be Tai Chi that's never been seen before and never will again.

That's expected of us, actually. There's no other way to claim our place in the lineage because ours is a lineage of lions.

APPENDIX A

Forty-Nine Principles of Tai Chi Awareness and Movement

<u>Attaining the View</u>

1. Eighty Percent Effort
2. Drop Down
3. Unhurriedness
4. Relaxation
5. Open Awareness
6. Balanced on One Leg
7. Bend the Knees
8. Buddha Belly, Buddha Breath
9. Vertical Spine
10. Body as Seaweed
11. Arms Spread, Elbows Down
12. Airy Hands
13. Distant Gaze
14. Elongate the Body
15. The Circle
16. Less is More
17. The Inner Glow

Grounding Our Practice

18. Horse and Rider
19. The Root
20. The Other
21. Front Foot Straight, Rear Foot Out
22. Knee Behind Toes
23. Foot and Knee Always Agree
24. Dripping Foot
25. Empty Foot, Move Foot, Fill Foot
26. Feet Come Together
27. Establish Rear Foot First
28. Foot Pivots on Heel
29. Shoulders Turn Foot
30. Control Hip Elevation
31. Tuck the Tailbone
32. The Empty Bowl
33. Hand at Hip, Hand at Shoulder
34. Hands Below Eyes
35. Level Shoulders
36. Tongue at Roof of Mouth
37. Left Side, Right Side
38. The Nine Directions

Coming to Life

39. Commitment
40. Shared Gestures
41. The Golden Thread
42. The Swan
43. Twist the Spine
44. First Do the Opposite
45. River or Mountain
46. The Colossus
47. Now Yielding, Now Powerful
48. Send the Chi
49. Audacity

Appendix B

The Yin-Yang Circle

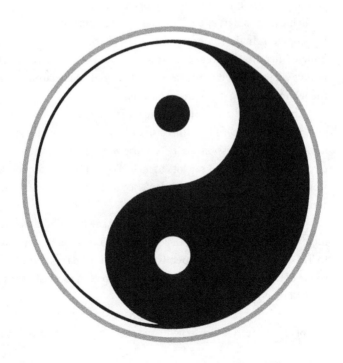

Appendix Z

We've a bit of room here at the end of the book for tying together loose ends and dangling one or two fresh ones. First I'd like to suggest to you that Tai Chi is an adaptogen. Think ginseng, an herbal medicine that's smart enough to adapt to each person and situation it encounters. In the same way, Tai Chi has been received and interpreted differently by every culture and century it's passed through, always adapting itself to the needs of the people it encounters—all the while retaining its essential nature.

There's a tendency, I think, once we've discovered something personally meaningful, to draw a small circle around it and say it's limited to *that* expression alone. To those who'd like to draw a small circle around Tai Chi, I say lots of luck. Tai Chi has been a rolling stone since its inception, and I don't see it slowing down anytime soon.

When people ask me what Tai Chi is, I say it's difficult to hit a moving target. Ultimately, it depends on who you are. People come to Tai Chi from every perspective and cultural background and shade of need. Still, it's pretty accurate to say that most of us enter Tai Chi through one of four doorways:

The original port of entry was the martial arts door. Tai Chi was first of all an effective way to fight, and that's how a lot of people still view it. Young men, in particular, are drawn to Tai Chi's competitive, athletic side. That's door number one.

Beginning in the middle of the last century, a huge wave of practitioners came along with no interest in pugilism at all. For them, Tai Chi was a way to hang onto your health in an increasingly stressful world. That would be door number two: holistic health.

And some come to Tai Chi for beauty's sake alone. For them, door number three is personal artistic expression.

The fourth doorway, my own, is something of a mystical/alchemical portal. I see Tai Chi as an enlightenment technology, a means of blending our outer selves, our personality selves, back into our original design, thereby discovering relevance and native joy.

The mystical/alchemical roots of Tai Chi are very deep, going back to old Taoist practices of breath, visualization, and purposeful movement, today known as Qigong—unquestionably the mother of Tai Chi. And the father? The father practice, developed in the Buddhist Shaolin temple, was a vigorous discipline now referred to as Kung Fu.

If your mother is Taoism and your father Buddhism, how can you not be a spiritual practice? Yet it becomes necessary to point this out because of the great pains the Maoists took last century to erase the spiritual side of Tai Chi.

So, door number four.

The thing is, no matter the doorway by which we enter Tai Chi, we wind up in the same room. We receive all the benefits. (Less so, perhaps, with the martial arts part because we really have to toil to become effective fighters using Tai Chi; that said, self-defense begins with being solid on our feet and aware of what's going on around us, and that comes with even casual Tai Chi practice.)

Finally, it's not for me or anyone else to tell you what Tai Chi is. Once you open this stuff up in your life, Tai Chi will become whatever you're lacking. That's why I call it an adaptogen.

We're very diverse in Tai Chi, and I say it's okay for us to be diverse. We should all feel good about our lineage, and our bodies and personal needs and interests. It's all Tai Chi, and it all works, and it's all deeply honorable.

But here's where I add my little bit. It's all Tai Chi as long as it occurs largely within the envelope of Tai Chi's underlying principles. See the above book. Say what you will, there is a specific way human movement and awareness are designed to operate. What we're doing is discovering and falling back on that design.

Next, more on relaxation.

In the following section, I want to really focus on becoming radically soft in our Tai Chi. That's where we go time and again because that's where self-transformation lies. In *radical* softness.

Core Tissues and Core Issues

As we learned in the text, if we want to find the really deep places in our Tai Chi, it's all about opening our awareness to ever finer degrees of experience. Where do we find those ever finer degrees? We find them in the *feelingness* of the body. The body has such incredible connectivity that I don't even know how to talk about it. The body is registering impressions outside its own boundaries. It's noticing things it can't possibly even know. That's its design. At which point, the term *body* doesn't even serve anymore.

Another way to say it is: the experience stream is so rich with information that we have to route most of it to our subconscious mind or we'd find it impossible to cross a street. We'd be incapable of focusing on anything. But all that information is still being received, and it's still becoming part of us, and it's our basis of intuitive decision-making.

Even the term *subconscious* needs re-examining. What is it about the subconscious that makes it so subconscious? It's that our attention is elsewhere. We're busy punching in a long phone number, so we're temporarily unavailable to probably 99.999999999% of the experience stream. Once we're off the phone, that number drops several decimal places. Once we're lying down in a dark, quiet room, it drops a lot more. Under hypnosis, we're able to access all kinds of information we'd otherwise consider unavailable. So there's no clear demarcation between available and unavailable content.

When we do Tai Chi, we're intentionally expanding our sphere of experience, claiming more and more of the subconscious as conscious. We're present and noticing. We're feeling. We're riding the experience stream like a cresting wave.

If we're really, really soft.

As we've discussed, softness begins with dropping down into the body and softening until all our inner bells are free to ring in resonance with the ambient music of the moment. It begins with dropping the shoulders and letting the belly sag forward, of course. And then it gets into dealing with our core tissues and core issues, which is a process I call *dropping the inner guard.*

Let's talk about that. Boxers are coached to never drop their guard, and I think we all absorb that lesson pretty early in life. You and I unconsciously tighten certain places as though we're expecting a sucker punch. Over time, this practice results in a tough, de-sensitized body. Now we're largely removed from the experience stream, which means our intuition is unavailable, plus our chi is all fouled up, so sooner or later someone hangs a diagnosis on us.

By the way, what is a diagnosis? I'll tell you what a diagnosis is. A diagnosis is a group of symptoms that's been seen before. What doctors do is take that cluster of symptoms and attach a name to it—usually an intimidating Latin name—and we're told quite soberly that we *have* something. I'm not sure how different that experience is from going to a fortune-teller and hearing that there's a curse on us, but the end result is the same: our power and our money wind up in the hands of the expert. Here's my advice the next time someone tries this on you: laugh. Over your shoulder as you walk out the door.

A group of symptoms may kill you. A diagnosis definitely will.

If you look beneath just about any group of symptoms, what you'll find is not a disease but a pattern of habitual tightness—which brings us back to dropping the inner guard. I'm speaking from experience here.

For many years I dealt unsuccessfully with a phantom heart problem before discovering that I was carrying an inner shield around my heart. If you or a loved one is experiencing phantom heart issues, listen in.

The thing to understand about the chest is that its bone structure is not at all static but composed entirely of moveable parts. The chest is designed to move *a lot*, especially to expand and contract freely with the breath. A tight, constricted chest limits the breath and oppresses the heart, making it feel cramped and under-oxygenated. That can very easily lead to symptoms of angina and elevated blood pressure.

My chest was so tight it almost didn't move at all. I'm talking about bricks and mortar. I suspect this happens to a lot of us when we're very young: we discover that the world is a hurtful place, so we build a shield around our hearts. It's an unconscious act that's intentional all the same. Finally, three years ago my acupuncturist Patricia said, "Your chest doesn't move. Did you know that? Your chest needs to move when you breathe. Otherwise you're not nourishing your heart and liver." Obediently I tried to expand my chest when inhaling. I couldn't. It didn't budge.

So I went to bodywork guru Ana, and we went to work on the problem. Ana was amazed at how impenetrable my chest was. It would take her half an hour of hard work to achieve a partial opening in my chest, and then the shield would repair itself in a matter of hours.

This thing was serious about its work.

It should go without saying that this kind of physio-emotional healing requires everything we can throw at it: talk therapy, nutritional therapy, body work, energy work, whatever you've got. I went at the shield from various angles, chipping away as best I could for a year or so, but there was little in the way of results.

I *had* to get rid of that thing. It was literally suffocating me. Once becoming aware of the shield, I understood where my phantom heart issues were coming from. My heart was constantly sore and exhausted from working in such cramped quarters. There was almost always a black sensation at the center of my chest that said *not enough oxygen here.* Those feelings had been there for a long time, and there'd been a couple of scary episodes, too. But the medical doctors had shrugged and said I was just experiencing a little stress.

As though that won't kill you.

To their credit, the alternative practitioners I consulted spent some time helping me focus on my emotional issues, but I wasn't able to find any traction until Patricia noticed that my chest wasn't moving. Not that I was able to do much about it once I knew. With Ana's help, yes, I could free up a little space but only temporarily.

Finally came a day when I was pretty much at wit's end. I was really flagging and out of ideas, and I fell on my bed and opened my mouth, and out came a sound. I suppose it was what people call *toning.* I'd never been taught how to tone, but suddenly this long, extended C# *aum*-type sound came out of me. It vibrated every bone and joint in my body but especially those of the chest. I knew that my body was taking over. It wasn't saying please anymore.

I lay there and toned for a full hour. I did the same thing the next day and the thirty-nine days after that, all the while telling my chest that it was okay to open now. I also did visualization and tapped my EFT points and repeated Ascension affirmations, and just generally hit that damn shield with everything I could think of, and I think those forty days made a difference. I know I felt much better after each session, and I hoped that the underpinning of the shield might be starting to break apart.

Still, nothing dramatic.

Fast forward to June of this year, nearly three years after beginning work on the shield. The full moon was in the east window of my living room. The lights were off. I was alone, half-reclined on the sofa, adrift in cricket song and moon glow.

All at once, for some reason I sensed a lot of power. The moment was extraordinarily dense with it. In particular I felt the power of my own will and knew that I could accomplish pretty much anything I wanted to do. Without giving it any thought, I reached down and touched my chest. I thanked the shield for all it had done. I said I no longer required its services, and I sent it away. I knew I'd never see it again.

Next morning, I had *breasts*. Not as pronounced as those of a woman, I'm happy to report, but my chest absolutely looked like that of some other person. It was fluffy. It was dual. And it *moved*. At the center of my chest, for the first time in memory, was a very distinct hinge joint that opened and closed with the slightest breath. I couldn't stop staring at it.

Or at my breasts.

Fast-forward to this very afternoon. I'm at my desk. Again the moon is full. It's been four months since I sent the shield away. It hasn't come back. The black sensation at the center of my chest is gone. My heart feels safe and content.

I think a lot of us are carrying around shields that we don't know about, and a lot of those shields involve the chest. As a culture, we are heart-sick. There's a veritable Long March of Americans trudging from doctor to doctor with very real chest symptoms, *very* real concerns, only to be told there's nothing wrong. Hopefully those people eventually learn of old emotional issues that concern their hearts.

Big-ass surprise, right? Take ten people off the street and you've got nine and a half with emotional issues around the heart. Finally, with luck along comes someone like Patricia (Patricia Campuzano, now retired), who's present enough to see what's right in front of her eyes.

The chest *has* to move. The lungs need to expand completely and not at the expense of the poor heart. If yours feels sore and oppressed and oxygen-deprived, it probably *is* sore and oppressed and oxygen-deprived. Go to work. Examine your posture. Spread your shoulders and lift your sternum and relax all the voluntary muscles you can. Then start working on your deep issues around safety and belongingness in this very difficult world.

I pass this story along because it's so easy to assume that our body is relaxed when it isn't relaxed in the slightest. I pass it along because core tissues and core issues can be successfully resolved *by ourselves* once we know what we're looking at. I tell this story so people will understand what a real healing curve may look like: slow and tedious with many fits and starts. The older the problem, they say, the more time and work that may be required to reverse it.

But notice the word *may*. Sometimes a miracle falls from the sky. You just say, "Please, God, unlock my chest," and it unlocks. That really happens, and it may happen for you. But I had to put in three years of work before my miracle fell from the sky.

Still, it fell. So persevere. Believe in your very real ability to call healing to yourself.

I once attended a seminar where the facilitator asked for a volunteer with some kind of movement restriction. A woman stood up and said she couldn't lift her right arm. After demonstrating her restriction, the woman was told to close her eyes and visualize her right arm rising straight into the air. Then she was told to open her eyes and raise her actual arm straight up in the air. And she . . . opened her eyes and raised her right arm straight up in the air. I loved the look on her face.

We are very funny creatures, you and I. We go around with our heads full of ideas about what reality can and can't do, and it's a bunch of hooey. You and I are magical beings. That's the long and short of it.

I attended another presentation where a volunteer from the audience lost twelve pounds of bodyweight sitting in a chair for five minutes. You should've been there. The demonstration was conducted at a university, and a professor from the physics department did the weighing with his own old-fashioned mechanical scale. The audience was blown away. *How* does a man lose twelve pounds sitting in a chair for five minutes? I'll tell you how. Everyone present spent the whole five minutes visualizing that exact outcome.

You and I seem to be onto something here, and here's what we seem to be onto: the body is always listening and responding. Reality itself listens and responds to what consciousness is looking at.

Want a good read? Find a copy of *101 Miracles of Natural Healing* by Luke Chan. It's a hundred one personal accounts of miraculous healings that occurred at an experimental hospital in Beijing. I attended a lecture by Mr. Chan in which he described that hospital. Every patient there had three things in common: they had been sent home to die, they didn't want to die, and they were willing to work.

All were taught a simplified form of Qigong which they practiced as a group eight hours each day. The other hours, they rested and encouraged one another. One by one, those people got up and went home. They literally picked up their beds and booked out of there.

Actually, there were two such hospitals in China, and their success was so phenomenal that the government shut them down. When people start discovering their own power . . . well, you finish the sentence. Anyway, my point isn't that Qigong is magical, nor is it that those two hospitals were magical. My point is that those hundred one people were magical. And so are you.

THE FASCINATING FASCIA

We can't really talk about softening the body without getting into the *fascia*, or the microfascial network, to be exact. That's a netting of fibrous tissue much like what plants use to hold themselves upright. You and I have an enormous wrap-around of that same kind of fiber beneath our skin. Otherwise we'd be amoebas. All our internal organs would be down around our knees. Fascia is what gives us our shape by not letting the body expand in certain ways. Think support pantyhose beneath your skin.

While it willingly stretches to allow the joints to move as intended, the fascia doggedly resists any movement that appears threatening. Fascia is feisty. Rubbed the wrong way, it tightens up and remains tight until the perceived threat has passed.

Where we get into trouble with the fascia is when some kind of traumatic event occurs. When we experience a shock of some kind, be it an automobile accident or a robbery, every part of the body is instantly notified by messenger chemicals in the bloodstream, and every part of the body reacts in its own way. The fascia reacts by tightening up, which is well and good, to a point. It provides us a bit of armor in a vulnerable moment.

But (and this goes for all the connective tissues of the body), what if we have trouble getting past our moment of trauma? The accident or robbery may be over in a matter of seconds, but emotionally it may still be with us a week later, or a month later, or a decade later. The body may keep reacting as though the event is happening now. We can have a bicycle accident when we're eight years old and still carry the injury in our microfascial tissue when we're eighty-eight.

The fascia remembers.

The good news is, it also learns. We can calm ourselves down and change the chemical messages moving through our blood-stream. We can pass old traumas out of our tissues.

Again, you and I are magical creatures. And it's just how things are set up. Either I'm badly wrong or it's impossible to have a question and not have the answer appear in the air all around us—and in every cell of the body—before we've had time to complete the question. Answers are drawn to questions through the information network I refer to as the inner glow, and our task is to become so transparent to that process that it registers in us as personal information.

Which brings us back to Tai Chi. Our daily movement practice is about a lot of things but none quite so much as this: becoming alert enough *and* soft enough for the obvious to penetrate. Just the obvious, not secrets on a scroll in some cave. Not special instructions channeled from a hovering spaceship—we don't need that. We're just talking about information that's readily available to anyone. We're just learning to become really, really good at noticing. That begins with alertness, but noticing alone doesn't get us very far without softness.

Which brings us back to the fascia. And the ligaments, and the tendons, and the core muscles of the body. It brings us back to every-thing we have that's capable of locking up and locking down.

Maybe you're really good at unknotting your tight spots while doing your daily Tai Chi. Great. Personally, I have to take it to the floor.

Getting Down and Dirty
with Floor Work

Some tight places in the body don't respond to nicey-nice. When I need to go into those really fearful places and coax them open up, it's not enough to send a brief mental suggestion. I have to really focus. I have to use my hands and my intention, and work very carefully, and that usually means going to the floor. It means using the floor's surface and my posture to isolate those knots and support them while they feel their way toward release.

When we're positioned on the floor just right, we can gently feel our way into where the problem lies. Then we lean into that spot just a little—not stretching it but simply opening a dialogue with it. We're applying just enough pressure to find those places in our attention, then we're letting our attention do the work.

We don't stretch, is the thing, we *elongate*. We use suggestion to release the tension from the center of the tissues and let those tissues expand naturally from their center. Outside force just causes more fear and more constriction. Never force. Cajole.

Everything I pretend to know about elongating is by way of aforementioned "bodywork guru Ana," who is Ana Maria Munoz Montero of Santiago, Chile. Ana's work is informed by the teachings of Gerda Alexander, the inventor of Eutony. The starting point in Eutony, as in Tai Chi, is respecting the intelligence of the body. Is there habitual tightness in a certain place? There's a reason for that!

We never *bull* our way into a tight place but initiate a co-equal conversation with the body.

There are some really tangy stories I could relate concerning Ana's work—surgeries averted, lifelong issues cured in a single session, that kind of thing, but I can only speak with authority of my own experience, so. . . .

Earlier this year, I appeared in Ana's studio with lower-back pain. I'd had a bunch of workmen in my house all day for weeks. Of *course* my body was tied up in knots. Ana had taught me how to work on myself when my lower back was absorbing stress, but this time I was getting nowhere fast.

Ana didn't even look at my back but had me lie face-up on the mat while she explored my chest. "Feel this," she said, moving my hand to my left ribcage. "Now feel this." Ana moved my hand to the right ribcage. "What do you notice?"

I'm not very smart in these things, but it was impossible to miss the fact that the left ribcage was much higher than the right. On my right side, the ribs were relaxed and spread out more or less as they should be. The left ribcage was so narrow and contracted that it jutted forward one or two inches beyond the right. I couldn't believe I hadn't noticed.

We're the last ones to see our own distortions. But once we're pressed against the floor, they tend to show up. Now we're able to use our hands and the pressure of the floor to gently go into those areas.

Next Ana told me to compare the left and right sides of my pelvis. Again I was shocked at the difference. My left side was really shrunken. Measured from the pubis to the outer tip of the hip, the left side was a good two inches shorter than the right. And we're talking about a very skinny body here. My hips measure (using a measuring tape now) eleven inches across, bony nub to bony nub. That day, they were nine inches wide: five and a half on the right, *three* and a half on the left. That sounds more like a Barbie than a human being.

But not for long. Ana applied some gentle shaking and coaxing, and minutes later the left side of my body had opened out dramatically, becoming observably broader than the right.

(Later she would work on the right side, equalizing everything, but Ana considers her work to be more instructional than remedial; she wants clients to learn to see their own distortions and work on them themselves, so she first releases one side of the body and has the client observe the difference between left and right, then releases the other side and has the client observe again.)

We are shape-shifters. That's the message here. The body is incredibly amorphous and responding constantly to what's going on within us and around us. Never let a doctor tell you that something has to be ripped apart and sewn back together "right." You can coax that same body part back into proper position in less time than it takes to talk about it. The body has a natural self-adjust impulse. All we have to do is learn how to induce that impulse.

Personally I find that really exciting.

"It's about your left side," observed Ana. I found that surprising, as my pain was centered on the right side of my lower back. Continuing down my body to the upper legs, Ana had me observe the *kwa* on either side, the folds where the thighs meet the body. It took a full minute of probing with my fingertips, but finally I noticed that the left side felt denser and tougher than the right. Ana showed me a knot in the fascia on the left side measuring two inches across. As she worked on dissolving that knot with her fingers, she asked whether I felt any kind of emotional charge in that place.

For a couple of minutes, I didn't. Slowly though it came to me that I was experiencing the presence of my late step-grandfather, someone I'd been close to as a child. It was as though I simultaneously smelled him, saw him, and heard his voice—only the impressions were emerging not from my thought-memories but from the tissues Ana was massaging. I was re-experiencing how my step-grandfather had moved: slowly and bent, yet with what seemed a sense of gusto.

As Ana worked, I re-experienced how he had always risen from the sofa with a theatrical groan. I recalled, too, the truss often left hanging on a doorknob in the bathroom. I remembered being called out, at age four or five, for mimicking the movements and groans of old people. "You stop acting like an old man!" I was told sharply. "You are a child!"

Who knows what mannerisms we pick up from others as small children? Who knows how much "hereditary illness" is actually hereditary ways of holding ourselves? What did my memories of a long-dead relative have to do with the knot on the left side of my body? I'll probably never know exactly, nor do I need to. I just breathed there and let the impressions move through me, and within minutes the lump began coming apart.

Next Ana focused my attention on the groin area inside each thigh: "Do you feel a difference between left and right?" It seemed to me that the left side was contracted. Shorter and tougher. Ana's fingertips pressed into that tissue, and she asked if I felt a response in my right lower back. I did. She explained that the two areas were connected between the legs by the muscle known as the psoas major. "Do you see now where your back pain is coming from?"

Call me a genius. I saw the connection. My lower-right back problem had nothing to do with my lower right back. It had everything to do with the huge contractions on the left side of my body. All the surrounding joints and tissues had literally gone out of their way to compensate, distorting the whole posture. Finally there came a breakdown. As always, it occurred at the weakest link in the chain. For me that was the lumbar.

After releasing both sides of my body, Ana withdrew to a chair and dictated certain movements (diagonal leg extensions) for me to do while lying on my back with legs raised. Instantly the first attempt took me into a painful spasm, and my whole body contracted horribly. "The least strength possible," coached Ana, meaning I was to use as little muscular force as possible while still accomplishing the movements.

After a few minutes of cursing my fate and all things Chilean, I found that if I proceeded very, very slowly I could work around the tender area. That was an important discovery because the pain and cramping were exhausting me far more than the actual movements. The movements were easy. (Tai Chi practitioners take notice: fatigue comes not from what we do but from our resistance to what we do.)

Encouraged, I delved deeper into this nebulous idea of selective muscle use. It was amazing. Just by being more gradual and intentional about which muscles I chose to contract, I could accomplish the assigned movements without difficulty. It was actually a little spooky because I wasn't consciously choosing which muscles to use, so much as *willing* it. I was soft-focusing my attention on the general area and intending, and the body was taking care of the details. Trust was involved. Trusting my body.

After a few minutes, I was extending my legs effortlessly and painlessly. It seemed they were moving themselves while I watched from a comfortable distance.

Something else interesting: I was seeing into how often, and how needlessly, I was tightening the area of the groin, particularly the psoas major. I was in the habit of tightening that area no matter the nature of my movement—as the previous week of torment had amply pointed out, since every movement I'd attempted had resulted in a painful contraction.

What were Ana's exercises showing me? That I was using my body fearfully, especially during really stressful periods in my life. Now I was seeing into that whole syndrome and realizing that, once aware, I could use my body in a completely different way.

"Good," said Ana. "Now, taking your time, when you're ready, stretch and stand up."

I *bounded* up, delighted to discover that my back pain was completely gone. Ana had me walk around the room while paying attention to the areas that had previously been tight. Everything Ana does is intended to focus you on the difference between being tight and being loose. Again, noticing.

Ana is a great example. She's been working on herself for so long that, in the middle of eating a sandwich, she'll suddenly exclaim, "Oh! My L5 just fell into place. It's been a little out all day." That's what we want. To become so aware of our inner places and inner spaces that we know right away when something's off. Most of us spend our days in a trace of numbness, of habitual ignorance, but we weren't designed to be that way. We've learned it, and we can learn differently.

At the end of my session, Ana gave me some exercises to do as homework—basically the same ones I'd just done. That's the *work* part of floor work. It's all on you. You created the problem. Go create the solution. The good news is: there's not a single one of us who can't do this kind of self-work and benefit from it enormously. The somewhat less good news is: nothing in our culture has prepared us to work on ourselves. We are taught to be dutiful consumers, and it's exactly this attitude that has us so goddamn numb and dependent and ill.

The back's better. Thanks for asking.

Actually there's one more twist to the story, and I'd like to share it. Before emerging from my adventure of the workmen and the shrunken left side, things took a really ghastly turn, to the point where even I could see it clearly. It looked like someone had sawed me in half and put the two parts back together wrong. My gut was *straddling* the point of my left hip. My torso was offset to the left by about four inches.

Somehow I wasn't in pain, but I knew it would only be a matter of time. For a few days, Ana and I worked in vain to convince my midsection to go back to its proper place. Finally a solution appeared out of left field.

I say out of left field because it was a flash of lightning, here and gone, but in that brief moment a window of opportunity opened and I was able to dart through. As in my earlier story, that window opened while I was sitting alone in the dark, this time without a moon in the window. It was just starlight and crickets and me.

As before, I noticed a lot of power in the moment. I felt clarity and unanimity, and I knew that I could say something to myself and it would be heard. So, there in my chair, I straightened my posture and pulled myself tall, and released my tension into the earth and said to myself, "This is how we are from now on. Vertical. Symmetrical. Relaxed. Open. Happy." For good measure, I repeated those words a couple of times while envisioning the posture I wanted and tapping my EFT points.

A few minutes later, I got up and checked myself in the mirror. My hip was back in place. Five months later, it's still in place.

We are mysterious creatures, you and I, and our healing paths don't always follow straight lines. There are unexpected turns along the way, and it pays to be alert to those flashes of lightning, those momentary windows of opportunity. To that end, you might really consider spending some time sitting alone in the dark, or near-dark. Sound depressing? It's not. Sound like sensory deprivation? It's quite the opposite. Electric lights conceal more than they reveal.

I might not have stumbled on that realization had I not done a lot of camping over the years, and fifteen years living off-grid. I've developed the habit of squaring everything away before nightfall then sitting and letting the darkness enfold me. I've learned that night is not for doing but for feeling. I've learned that when we insist on expanding the day into night through the use of (violent!) electric lights, enormous opportunities come and go without our even knowing about them.

The Chinese talk about *wu wei*, or doing nothing. If we're present and softly alert and paying attention to what's rolling in and what's rolling out, doing nothing becomes a very legitimate enterprise. Call it meditation if that makes you feel better. I call it sitting there.

ANOTHER STORY YOU CAN SCARCELY BELIEVE!

Another cautionary tale about getting myself in a jam then getting myself out again (it's the way I learn; I think it may be the way we all learn): I was traveling long-distance by bus a few days before Christmas—never the best of ideas—and in the general bedlam I neglected to buy loss insurance for my bag. That turned out to be a serious lapse because I'd packed some important things inside, including about three thousand dollars' worth of new electronic gear.

I know. I know.

But what could go wrong? Each time I changed buses, I watched them load my bag, actually a large cardboard box, into the cargo bay before I boarded. But late that night, just before I crossed from Texas into Mexico, I discovered that my bag was gone. It had evidently been wrongly unloaded somewhere in the night and likely thrown onto a bus to Bangor, for all the bus company could tell me.

I was also told that the company's system for rerouting lost luggage was basically nonexistent. The box *could* eventually turn up there in Laredo, I was told, but likely not before mid-January. Even then, I'd have to be physically present to claim the box or it would be shunted off to a warehouse somewhere in the Midwest that they no longer had a phone number to.

Nice.

My choices came down to: (1) I could live at the Laredo bus station from that moment forward, personally checking the cargo bay of each bus that arrived; or (2) I could surrender to my exhaustion and cross into Mexico without my belongings, meaning I would definitely never see them again. The bus people really, *really* didn't care one way or the other. Thanks for traveling Greyhound.

Well, here it was midnight and I hadn't slept in a couple of days nor eaten anything resembling food, so the first thing I had to do was get a hold of myself. In an angry daze I staggered around defunct downtown Laredo until finding a place to more or less eat and hydrate. Then I settled onto a park bench and said to myself, "Okay, here's the deal. I can go on being astonished and appalled, or I can bring that box to me. If I want the latter, I have to really, really focus. The exhaustion and indignation—have to go. The sense of powerlessness definitely has to go."

There on the park bench, I gradually calmed my breathing and dropped my attention into my body. I sensed my box sitting right in front of me.

I saw the extra packing tape I'd swaddled it in. I read the name and address I'd written in black marker. I smelled the cardboard and the yellow nylon rope I'd tied securely around it. I felt that rope dig into my palms as I lifted the box from the cargo hold of an idling bus. I inhaled the exhaust fumes as I dragged it along the rough asphalt in the chilly night. I felt my weary exultation as I thanked every star in heaven. My belongings had come back to me! I spent exactly fifteen minutes living that reality.

Then, worry free, I got up and returned to the bus station.

My box wasn't on the next bus that arrived, nor was it on the tenth or twelfth. But sometime very late that night, just as I'd envisioned it would, my box appeared in the cargo hold of an idling bus, and I dragged it away, thanking every star in heaven.

Can I prove that I brought that box back to me? Can you prove I didn't?

People Be Like Trees

Earlier we mentioned becoming a different visual statement through Tai Chi, and I'd like to go back to that idea for a moment. I used to spend a lot of time in the forest with a knowledgeable woodsman named Frank Troskey, who taught me a lot about trees and how they adapt. "There's a tree that grows in an open space," he said, "and there's the same tree growing in a tight spot."

They become very different visual statements, is the idea. In an open space, a tree expands laterally and develops a strong root system. That tree is able to match its design, and it has a chance for a long, prosperous life.

The same tree growing in a dense forest becomes narrow and tall, shooting skyward as fast as it can. The latter situation, said Troskey, doesn't allow for very good development. Should some of the surrounding trees die or be cut down, that tree wouldn't be able to stand for long. The first windstorm would likely take it out.

Likewise, you and I are greatly influenced by our circumstances. An open, friendly environment encourages us to expand and develop strong limbs and roots, and we have a chance for a long, prosperous life. We match our design.

A cramped, threatening environment, on the other hand, makes us narrow and competitive; we pull in our posture, we pull in our energy, and we project ourselves forward in time. That's not very good

development. Should our outer situation change suddenly, we're ex-
posed for what we have become, and the first real storm may take us
out. We don't match our design. We just match our circumstances.

Take a look at the people around you. It's often easy to see at
a glance the kind of circumstances a person has experienced. We
become different visual statements. But here's the thing. We aren't
trees. We have legs. We can go someplace else. We can give our children a better opportunity to fully develop than we ourselves may
have had.

Get out of town.

Here's the other thing. Even if we didn't have that exquisite
freedom, even if, heaven forbid, we were forced to live in a prison
cell—we could *still* decide to open out our posture, and open out our
energy, and open out our breath, and pull ourselves tall, and drop
our tension, and we could *still* match our ideal design.

That's the power of Tai Chi.

HANDS CIRCLE UP, HANDS CIRCLE DOWN

This could almost be another principle of Tai Chi movement, but we'll leave it as an observation. Most Tai Chi moves develop from either of two basic patterns: the hands are circling up the center of the body, or the hands are circling down the center of the body. A good example of the former is Wave Hands in Clouds. If the hips and shoulders were held stationary (as they shouldn't be), the hands would make small circles that rise up the center of the body.

We all know how easily this move segues into Single Whip. Why? Because Single Whip is another move that uses the same up-the-center principle. Notice, too, how easily we can go from Wave Hands into Hold the Ball, or the Circle Down part of Frog Kick or of Close Tai Chi.

Likewise, there's a family of moves that flow from circling the hands down the center of the body. Brush Knee Push is one. White Crane Spreads Wings is another, as is Needle at Bottom of Sea.

When combining moves into a sequence, we often experience difficulty when transitioning from one of these families of moves into the other. How best to accomplish this kind of transition? Experiment.

Dogs, Cats, and Stance

Have you ever watched a dog or cat settle in for a nap? There's a lot of fussing about and circling and pawing and snorting and carrying on. What's all that about? Getting it right is what it's about. *Almost* right isn't good enough for a dog or a cat, and it shouldn't be good enough for you or me, either.

In Tai Chi, if the stance I'm settling into isn't quite right—stop the music. Nothing can go forward until my stance is right. I take the time to fix it. I interrupt the sequence, I interrupt the forward flow of time, I interrupt the moon's arc across the heavens, and I fix my stance. If that requires fussing about and circling and pawing and snorting—well, what else is the moment for? Either everything we're doing in Tai Chi is important, or none of it is.

Listen to me. No, really. Listen. *This* stance, this moment, this posture, is your last great stand on this beautiful Earth. That has to be the attitude. We are the Dog Soldier, and this posture sums up everything we've ever stood for, everything we cherish, everything we've ever dreamed to be true. We get it right if it takes all of today and half of tomorrow.

Do this and, I assure you, history will wait as long as necessary for you to array yourself exactly as you were designed to do. Why do I say that? For the simple reason that history *occurred* in order that you might now do what you were designed to do.

Be what you are, and do what you're doing.

Indulge me for another brief. I used to live with a couple of high-strung lapdogs. They weren't *my* high-strung lapdogs, I hasten to add. The point is, the experience provided an opportunity to learn something: how animals go about managing their stresses and frustrations. Now you get to learn it.

Each time something truly harrowing came up—which was about a dozen times a day—those dogs *threw* themselves upon each other with snarls and snaps and just the most awful behavior you're ever likely to see, or lapdog version of same. Still, I had to acknowledge that Li'l Bit and Katy were at least as intelligent as I insofar as stress management.

What was I doing with my stresses and frustrations? Dumping them straight into the shadow. I'm sure you know what I mean by that. When we humans feel something we don't wish to feel, we swallow it. We pretend it isn't there. The result? Our unexpressed feelings wind up in the tissues of the body, and we're well on our way to illness.

I believe that on some level Li'l Bit and Katy knew that. Every time those little dogs felt their bodies fill with anxiety, it *had* to come out. It had to be expressed as physical movement, and it didn't matter to them how it looked. So they "acted out." They used cathartic drama to drain their bodies of energy that couldn't express any other way. Those dogs never once harmed each other. It was pure Hollywood. And, as a result, they were clean little machines. Healthy and bright-eyed and shining in the moment.

Meanwhile, how was I doing? I was switching anti-depressants every few months. I was so full of repressed anger I couldn't even find it. Oh, but I was very well behaved.

My point? We humans experience lots of emotions and impulses we're unable to express, and those energies need to become physical movement and quickly. It can't wait till summer vacation. It can't even wait until the weekend. What we need is a daily conscious movement practice centered around feeling and allowing. We're allowing impulses to rise from our depths and express out as truthful movement. It doesn't have to be violent or dramatic. It becomes whatever it needs to be. We're just opening up a space.

One more doggie footnote and we'll be done. For now. Again, this concerns stance.

If you've ever gotten into a serious disagreement with a dog—I used to be a milkman, and I can tell you some stories—you know that dogs are expert at something martial artists call *distancing*. Moving forward and back. Dogs are built expressly for distancing. They set their hind legs behind them and their forelegs before them, and they hug the ground, and a swift kick has no chance at all of landing. Not that I would ever kick a poor helpless dog. Throwing an empty milk bottle works better.

We want that same distancing thing in our martial arts practice, and to that end we always set one foot to the fore and the other to the rear. Our hips, meanwhile, are lowered to the point where we can move in and out quickly. Plus we're shifting our bodyweight forward and back, now over the front leg, now over the rear, and we're re-positioning our feet, sliding to and fro, distancing ourselves as the moment requires.

Obvious? I suppose so, but when we're beginners, stance is such a static thing. We're just standing there. Properly understood, stance is a flowing thing.

That's true in our solo Tai Chi, and it's even more true when we're engaged in sparring. Once we have the basics of stance down, just what goes where, we need to drill moving forward and back, forward and back, sometimes stepping-through (alternating which foot is forward), sometimes sliding, sometimes springing. Should the opponent threaten us with a kick, we fade back just enough for the kick to spend itself in the air then instantly come forward with a counterattack before he can re-set himself. That's the basic riff of distancing.

Thanks to all the dogs and cats out there.

Really, when you think about it, four-legged animals have all the advantages. You and I, being so very vertical and having just two legs, are always in danger of going down. We have just one advantage over the quadrupeds: we're great conservers of energy. Quadrupeds burn a lot of energy just standing there, and running tires them very quickly. Great sprinters, quadrupeds, but not at all effective over a distance. They peter out.

Here's a question for you. Of all the animals in the world, how many can outlast a human over a long distance? The answer: not a single one. Eventually we run them all into the ground. Horses, greyhounds, cheetahs, everything. We are masters of stamina because we're masters of verticality.

Just wanted you to know.

I'm Better When I Move

Film buffs will recognize that quote from *Butch Cassidy and the Sundance Kid*. Robert Redford's character is trying unsuccessfully to shoot a tin can while standing still. Then he begins moving and shooting from a crouched position, and he hits the can several times, spins his pistol and holsters it, commenting, "I'm better when I move."

We're all better when we move.

In Chapter Three we considered the idea that movement connects us to truth in some kind of fundamental way, as though truth itself were in motion. Certainly I think our senses are more impressionable when we're in motion.

We know that water is very impressionable. (See the work of Masaru Emoto.) I recently read that water is more impressionable when moving, especially when moving in a circular manner. I don't know how true that is, but it got me thinking.

Upwards of seventy percent of the human body is water. So when we're doing Tai Chi, and we're describing circular movements, and our bodies are soft and receiving—shouldn't that do something? Shouldn't that imprint the water in our bodies with our intention and just our whole Tai Chi process?

Certainly something happens when we move.

There's a huge amount of research being done on water now, and it's impossible to say where it's all leading, but certainly I see water as a living creature that, like all living things, is either in a healthy or unhealthy state. And the closer we come to understanding the water in our bodies, the closer we may come to understanding ourselves.

Drink good water, the best you can get your hands on.

Move with awareness each day.

Eat your vegetables.

More on the Directions

We've talked about the importance of the eight directions in classical Chinese thought. We can choose how much to emphasize the directions in Tai Chi. One of the things I've done in the past is to begin and end class facing a certain way and say something like:

"We dedicate this class to *Chen*, the energy of the east and the birthplace of the sun. *Chen* is the place of beginnings and of possibilities. May we too live with passion and inspire in others the desire to live our highest, truest lives."

If this kind of thing interests you, here are a few words concerning each direction:

Kan, Energy of the North

The symbol of *Kan* is water, which falls to the lowest places of the earth and so nurtures all living things from below. May we too learn that, while there is a time to rise to the zenith, there is also a time to sink to the depths, as does sap sink to the roots of a tree in winter. Only through humility do we discover the strength to rise to our fullest potential.

Ken, Energy of the Northeast

Ken represents the mountain and the power of remaining still. There are times when even correct actions will not meet with success. At those moments, like the mountain, may we too know the wisdom of remaining still.

Chen, Energy of the East

Chen represents enthusiasm. The symbol of Chen is thunder, whose sudden appearance instills great excitement. May we too live with passion, inspiring in others the desire to live their highest, truest lives.

Sun, Energy of the Southeast

Sun represents the wind, the teacher of gentleness. Though the wind has great power, it willingly parts for the smallest tree. When the time comes for shaking loose the old and the lifeless, only then does the wind come with all its power. May we too learn to use our strength only when it serves the highest good.

Li, Energy of the South

Li represents fire and transformation. Just as the sun never ceases its work of transforming darkness into light, may we be the fiery alchemists of this world, working with great diligence until all is transformed into brilliance.

Kun, Energy of the Southwest

Kun represents the feminine, whose wisdom is to receive. May we too learn to listen, to absorb, and to accept with gratitude. We give thanks to the Earth, who is our mother, and to our birth mothers, and to every loving hand that has ever aided, that we may now aid others.

Tui, Energy of the West

Tui's gift is that of joy. Like a spring overspilling its banks, may we too be a source of joy to those around us. Like *Tui*, let us remember to laugh, never taking ourselves too seriously, ever creating yet mindful that we ourselves are created again each moment.

Chien, The Energy of the Northwest

Chien is the direction of creativity and of action. It represents the warrior spirit. When the moment comes for action, may we have the courage and decisiveness to throw aside caution and give ourselves completely to what must be done.

Wu Chi, Energy of the Center

We acknowledge the presence of *Wu Chi*, the primordial stillness at the center of all things. May we never lose our grounding in stillness, for it is the basis of all right action. May the infinite potential of *Wu Chi* be at the center of all we feel, think, and do.

ADD AND TAI CHI

Many people say Attention Deficit Disorder (ADD or ADHD) is nothing but a scheme by Big Pharma to put all our kids on drugs. I say it's more than that. Who knows what's causing the whole developed world to experience the current explosion of diseases and mental illnesses that never used to be a problem? But it's happening. I myself have had to deal with ADD symptoms all my life, and I can tell you it's real. Am I on drugs? No, I'm on Tai Chi.

Daily exercise is *highly* indicated for people with depression and ADD (which often appear in tandem). Exercise stimulates production of exactly the neurotransmitters people like myself tend to be short of. And it's a way of gaining traction, of breaking the downward spiral of "I can't get it together on any level." It just generally puts us on the good foot.

A personal Tai Chi practice goes even farther because it helps us find our own proper pace through life, our own way of focusing, our own way of meeting the world. Tai Chi helps us access our inner wells of motivation and inspiration. It calms us down and returns us to our center as does meditation, only it doesn't require sitting motionless for long periods of time (torture!).

There are a lot of misconceptions about ADD. People think you have to be hyperactive and disruptive in school. They think that without medication you're incapable of holding your attention still for more than a few seconds. Those things are completely untrue of me, and I'm sure they're untrue of millions of others with ADD.

Personally I just experience a lot of difficulty around doing certain things like picking up the phone or going to the grocery store. I can and have put off a necessary phone call for months, and it's not at all uncommon for me to eat the very last thing in the kitchen before going shopping. I thought I was just some strange variety of loser-head before someone suggested I answer a questionnaire about ADD. In my sixties I learned I'd "been ADD" my whole life.

Despite what you may have heard, many ADDers have excellent mental focus. We just need something worth focusing on. People like myself—and forgive me if I'm overgeneralizing, but I think this is true—despise the meaningless clutter and crapola of everyday life. We tend to be in escape mode, yes, but not because we're cowards or slackers. Maybe we're just smart. Maybe we're just sensitive to the fact that most of what's out there isn't worth the headache.

If ADDers tend to cling to the shadowed fringes of society—and we do—could it be that we're just highly uncomfortable around meaningless noise? Some New Agers go so far as to say ADDers are highly evolved beings.

I like that theory.

Certainly we are unique people who see the world in a unique way. That means people with ADD have something to offer—but first there's work to do. We have to get real about our strengths and weaknesses. We have to be clear about which outside influences are good for us and which aren't. We definitely need people around us who understand our ways and enjoy our company. People who just want to lecture? Let them go lecture each other. We feel bad enough about ourselves as it is.

If you, kind reader, have your own peculiar ways of seeing and being, and it's causing you problems, get checked out. For some people, medication evidently helps. But first of all, it's about getting on our own team. It's about becoming positive about ourselves and our funny, funny ways.

It's about getting on the good foot. And Tai Chi can really, really help with that.

The Handy Hand

Here's a practical tidbit you may enjoy. When we're talking about the particulars of a given Tai Chi posture, it can be helpful to use your own hand as a measuring device. As a common example, when the hand is lowered, the distance between the hand and the hip is usually stated as *one hand-width*. That means the width of the palm, including the thumb. That's a great way of saying it because bodies come in very different sizes, and hands tend to be proportional.

I also think in terms of *hand-span*, which is the maximum width of the hand from the tip of the extended thumb to the tip of the extended pinkie. We just open the hand as wide as we can, and there it is. I use this a lot in my Tai Chi because it gives me a quick way of checking certain points of posture, and it's a good teaching device because it applies equally to everyone.

As an example, when I bow, I position my hands a single hand-span away from my chest. When I'm in standing meditation posture (Stand Like a Tree), the distance is two hand-spans. As a general rule, I like to keep my hands between one and two hand-spans from my body.

Try it on for size.

The Rocking Chair

In Chapter Six, we talked about how we're always shifting the bodyweight in Tai Chi. That shifting can become very rhythmic and we experience what I call the rocking chair. We're literally rocking ourselves. The lower and wider the stance, the more pronounced the effect. Sometimes I emphasize that back-and-forth sway, making it very regular and soothing.

We can see it as a pendulum, speeding up as it plunges then slowing as it rises. A pendulum is actually motionless for a moment when it reaches the turning point. We too can slow the shifting of our bodyweight as we approach the high turning point. Then we gather speed once more as we drop our weight toward the center.

I find it interesting, as I go through a Tai Chi sequence, to isolate one leg in my awareness and see how that leg passes through its cycle of being filled and being emptied, being filled and being emptied. It's the Moon cycle. It's the Sun cycle. It's the everything cycle. At the same time, the other leg is cycling in *exactly* the same way in mirror image.

It's interesting to isolate one arm, one shoulder, whatever, in our awareness and follow it through a sequence of moves. Then see if the opposite side of the body is moving accordingly in counterpoint.

Experiment. Discover. Play. We want our Tai Chi to be a living, breathing organism, a bit different each moment and maybe strikingly different each year.

A Spirited Conversation
Among Myself

We've spoken of Tai Chi as sacred encounter. We've described it as a relationship workout. Certainly it is those things. There are conversations going on inside ourselves, as well, and these too are part of the dance. As we saw in Chapter Forty, our constituent parts are always dialoguing in Tai Chi, and that's true on levels we haven't even touched on.

In Tai Chi one body part is saying *hi* to another in passing, and the other is saying *hi* back. At the conclusion of Part Wild Horse's Mane, you've got one arm coming forward while the other is dropping to rest position. As the two arms pass each other, they share a gesture that suggests the combing of a horse's mane. (Imagine that the mane is draped over the forward forearm and wrist, while the fingers of the descending hand are the comb.)

That shared gesture can be celebrated or it can be entirely missed. I say, let's celebrate that. Let's not go to sleep on these moments. Tai Chi is about relationship. No relationship, no Tai Chi.

It helps if the two body parts *slow* just a little as they pass one another. Let them really feel one another's presence. The attitude and behavior of each should be affected by the presence of the other. Try it now and see for yourself. When the two hands are actively co-creating, it's a very different thing from the hands passing like ships in the night. Repeat this a few times and feel it from the perspective of each of your limbs in turn.

What's really intriguing is when one side of the body demonstrates a move for the other. Maybe one arm understands a certain move while the other arm doesn't get it. Arm A teaches arm B. That's more involved than it may sound because all the left-right stuff has to be flipped and the mental image reversed—and this generates growth on both sides of the brain. Meanwhile, we're watching all that happen, which is a *third* perspective.

Not long ago, I realized that my dominant (left) shoulder was always in charge of Single Whip, no matter the side I did it on. So I looked closely into that, and I determined that the *rear* shoulder should be the one in charge. The problem was, my recessive (right) side didn't know how to lead. So I let my dominant shoulder teach the recessive shoulder how that's done.

So now I'm watching this whole process, and one of my brains is talking to the other, and the other's saying *but how do you do that wrist thingie?* And the answer's coming back: *see? Like this.* And then it's: *but my wrist doesn't move like that. It was broken playing football, remember?* On and on.

You're witnessing all this, and information's crossing boundaries within yourself, and all this is registering in your greater awareness because you've learned how to notice. So now you've got new neural branching going on, and you know it because you're watching it branch. You're feeling it happen.

What's really interesting is when one of your brains says to the other *how exactly do you do that funny thing you do?* And the other brain replies *gee, I don't know. Let's watch and see.* Then the body performs the move, and *both* brains observe and discover the answer. What's going on, as I see it, is that the detailed information, the boilerplate, was long ago shunted off to the subconscious (whatever brain that is), and that information's floating back up, and now it's a three-way conversation. Four-way, actually, if you count yourself as witness.

Self is a complicated business. Really, I don't know how anyone can expect a professional career from any of us. We have all we can do just being somebody.

Vivaldi and Time

One recent morning I awoke in something of a dreamy state, and Vivaldi was on the stereo, and something came to me. A harpsichord and guitar were playing one of Mr. V.'s really bright and bubbly compositions, and it was hitting me just right, and I was surprised to find myself *exactly* on the pulse of the moment, right at the breaking edge of the event horizon, and I realized that until that moment I'd never really heard music. I'd never experienced it in its native state.

For me, music had always been something viewed through a five- to ten-second time frame, which I think is what most of us do: we consider each moment in the light of what came just before and what's likely coming next. That's how we follow the twists and turns of the melody line, and, if there are lyrics, the narrative line and rhyming scheme.

If the first line of the melody ends with an upturned note, one that dangles a question, we quite naturally expect the following line to pose a reply, ending on a downturned note that completes the thought. Alternatively, the second line may end with a minor-chord sidestep that delays the consummation of the melody; still, most composers provide a tidy conclusion every ten seconds or so, or the natives become restless. That's the game of melody, and of rhyme, and of lyric, and it requires an active attention span of five to ten seconds, which is where most of us are comfortable.

Even then, short-term memory is at best an eighteen-second proposition, and no matter how we strain we're rarely able to hold an entire five- or ten-minute composition in our minds. We've an eighteen-second window, tops, beyond which we're dealing with mental constructs. We're stepping back and comparing the piece as a whole to other compositions. We're constructing a model of the piece in our heads and referring to the model rather than to the actual experience. It's music as a mental exercise, which unfortunately is where most of us reside.

And yet!

Here was Vivaldi making *absolute magic* inside a time frame of about a fourth of a second. His notes came in spontaneous bursts, each a brilliant flash of light with only the scantest reference to past or future. I realized that my challenge as a listener wasn't to stretch my attention span longer so much as to collapse it into a singularity.

Lying on my bed in that dreamy state and listening to that piece took me to a place of—what can I say?—I found myself witnessing the creation of the universe in real time. I was seeing the instant-to-instant bubbling forth of divine exuberance into strutting form. Vivaldi, I realized, had witnessed that very thing, that very miracle, and had encoded it into the music I was witnessing.

Implicit order, I was being shown, is spun into packets so *very* tiny and fleeting they can only be kissed as they fly, can only be appreciated through a slit of time so vanishingly narrow it requires our very soul just to be with it for five seconds. To stay with it for ten requires the skills of a master surfer.

Which is where we circle back to Tai Chi. In our art, we are constantly challenged to ride the breaking edge of the moment, to stay upright on the board for one more instant, one more instant, to remain in the micro-moment despite the enormous longitudinal weight of context. Tai Chi beginners are always thinking ahead to the next move, the next series of moves, wearily smelling the oats in the barn, as the attention stretches thinner and thinner until it breaks and we collapse against the mental model rather than the actual experience.

It's called wiping out.

That's true of surfing, it's true of music, and it's true of Tai Chi. Neither you nor I are interested in mental models. We want to be burned clean by the fiery luminescence of the breaking moment, to be *right* there with Mr. V. making absolute magic inside a time frame of a fourth of a second.

Yes, we'd like to expand our attention longitudinally, to break through the eighteen-second wall, but the way we accomplish that is by *condensing* our attention into a singularity that can shoot through the eye of the needle and arrive at the flash-point of creation, the breaking edge of the event horizon, which unwinds and unwinds ceaselessly, carrying us along with it.

Do not surrender fiery Vivaldian luminescence to the dreary longitudinal frame. That's what the maestro whispered in my ear that sleepy morning. And it's what our Tai Chi whispers to us each moment.

Twenty Years of
Schooling and . . .

Once at a Yang-style workshop, I took advantage of a break to ask the instructor a question about a particular move in the Hundred-Ten. We were being taught a very odd embellishment on Wipe Tiger's Mouth that seemed to have no practical purpose. Not only that. It flew in the face of the principle River or Mountain.

Puzzled, I asked about it, and the instructor, a very knowledgeable master whom I respect completely, smiled and said, "It has no purpose. That variation was put in some time ago by a teacher who wanted all his students to be recognized as belonging to him. Now that it's in the lineage, we have to learn it."

Hmmm.

Later that day, I asked whether it's ever permissible for a mortal such as myself to make a change in how he performs the Hundred-Ten. The reply was, "Sure, after you've done it exactly as taught for twenty years."

Again, hmmm.

Maybe it's just me. But imagine some poor piano student being told he can create as much fresh, original music as he wishes—after putting in twenty years of only practicing scales. That probably wouldn't work for many developing musicians, and it didn't work for me as a developing practitioner of Tai Chi.

Personally, I cut the cord in my twelfth year of practice. At the same time, I began encouraging my students to experiment anytime they wished.

Listen, numbered sequences were invented by people exactly like you and me. The Twenty-Four-Movement Form, for example, is about as old and venerable as the Hula-Hoop. It was put together by a committee in 1957 by order of the Chinese government, which wanted a brief, lowest-common-denominator sequence that would simplify tournament judging. Most of the sequences circulating today have roughly the same pedigree.

I say it's the individual moves that count, not the way they're strung together. I have a vocabulary of thirty-six Yang-style moves, and I sequence them any way I please. Or not at all. Sometimes I devote an entire session to a single move, walking forward and backward, turning left and right, doing one-eighties, crabbing to either side. If the only contact we have with a move is its lone expression, often on *one* side of the body, as part of a memorized sequence—

Hmmm.

Mad Clothing, Fun, and Other Largely Forbidden Things

I say there are two kinds of martial artists: those who dress up and perform for the mirror, and those who lie about it.

Listen, the more fun we're having in our movement practice, the stronger it's becoming and the more powerfully it's going to impact our lives. Dress up. Perform for the mirror. Then lie about it.

If you've already installed a mirror where you practice, now go a little farther. Install good lighting. Try various set-ups until you find one that makes you look great. Indirect lighting is usually better, as are "warm"-colored bulbs. And you want light hitting you from two or more directions, which makes for flattering highlights, shadows, and even backlit effects.

Now find some fun threads. Maybe you look great in your same ol' Tai Chi uni. You probably don't. Now hit a few rummage sales, and don't be shy. Vests, capes, skirts, gowns, hats—bring a little of everything home and have a try-on party. Don't be afraid of colors you've never worn before. I find it's particularly fun to play with fabrics that drape and flow and sail in the wind. Once you know what looks interesting on you—what surprises you and brings out unexpected colors in your movements—design and sew your own outfits.

Does this idea sound totally inappropriate to you? Good! That means you really need to hear it. Loosen up, okay? Visit a troupe of belly dancers and see how they approach *their* movement practice.

See how much innocent fun they create with their outfits and their makeup and their big happy smiles. See, in particular, how *transformed by joy* they are by what they're doing.

Can you match that with what you're doing in your movement practice?

Belly dancers could perform those same movements in grey sweats or military uniforms, but they don't. Know why? Of course you know why. That kind of drab, serious clothing is a very poor match for the human spirit.

Anything begun with a grim attitude is wrong already. That includes your and my Tai Chi, my friend.

More Stupid Chi Tricks

Here's a stupid chi trick you may enjoy:

Find an overstuffed chair, seat yourself comfortably with your hands resting on the arms, and relax. Alternatively, you can place your forearms and hands on a tabletop. Either way, your fingers should be spread gently, including the thumb. Give yourself about a minute to settle into this posture, then another minute to notice the inner spaces of your body. You're not noticing the flesh so much as the space beneath the flesh, the space the body is written on. Just see what's there, without straining, making sure all the while that your hands are completely relaxed.

Once you have a general impression, a snapshot of that feeling, make one small adjustment. Reposition your thumbs, spreading them as wide as possible without introducing tension. That's probably about an eighty-degree angle. Now return your attention to the inner spaces of the body.

Notice any difference?

Many people find the difference nothing short of astonishing. Myself, I feel a portal yawning open at the junction of my thumb, flooding my whole body with light. It's said that every joint in the body acts as an energy portal, and when we open that joint, we open that portal.

Am I saying that every joint of the body should be wide open all the time? Not at all. The natural rhythm of everything, from micro-organisms to galaxies, is open/close. There's a time to open, there's a time to close, and there's a time when we're just somewhere in between. So we're not talking about the "proper" positioning of the thumb. We're acknowledging that there are no small things in the body, and so there are no small things in Tai Chi.

Another stupid chi trick, anyone?

Here's an energy experiment that involves the move Brush Knee Push. If you're not familiar with that move, just use the palm of either hand to very lightly push forward. You're imagining that you're sending positive energy to someone. If it seems easier, use a photo, or a stuffed animal, or anything else you choose, to represent the recipient.

In this particular exercise, we're sending energy out through the palm of the hand. What I do is germinate a loving thought in my heart and send it spiraling through the arm then out through the center of the palm—then through the air to the recipient. After a couple of minutes, you may feel something. This is a really simple technique, but it works every time, whether we feel something or not. And the positive energy arrives in us, as well. Again, what we put out is what we get.

As we've seen, we can also use visualization to pull energy into our bodies. In Chapter Forty-Eight, we discussed drawing chi from trees. I've received similar instruction for drawing energy from distant mountaintops, and even from the moon and stars. We just imagine that our arms and hands are long enough to reach those places. (Always ask permission first.)

There's no end to the stupid chi tricks we can do. In truth, the only stupid experiment is the one we don't try. Just keep it positive, and keep it simple, and it's all to the good.

And yet. Here's one caveat. Just because we may be a martial arts instructor, that doesn't mean we take it on ourselves to treat a specific ailment in someone's body. It's become trendy for martial arts instructors to rub their hands together and place them on anyone who complains of an ache or pain. Careful. That person may be experiencing too much chi in the affected area, not too little. Have you received training in energy diagnosis and healing? If not, go get some or it's hands-off.

Stranger's Face

When we go about relaxing the body in Tai Chi, you and I are apt to forget about the face. Oddly, we may not think of it as belonging to the body. It does, and the face accumulates and holds a lot of tension.

When we release the face in Tai Chi, we want to feel it fall. We want to feel it dripping off our chin and puddling at our feet. In Tai Chi, we want to become unrecognizable to ourselves. Who *is* this person doing my Tai Chi?

There've been many days when someone other than myself has done my fifteen minutes of Tai Chi. I drop my face, and my personality drains away, and all at once someone else is Parting Wild Horse's Mane. I feel some other person's features where mine used to be. It's often the same guy, a little Asian fellow with a short beard. I'm not complaining. That little guy's pretty good.

What we're doing is dropping the act. We're pulling the plug on *The Me Show, Starring Me*. Suddenly there's only consciousness and energy and expression. Whose no longer matters.

Specifically, let's make sure that the jaw is very loose and relaxed in our Tai Chi. For many of us, the jaw is active even when we sleep. We want that jaw to *sag*. When doing Tai Chi, I separate the upper and lower teeth while keeping the lips closed. (It's okay if the lips part a bit, as long as we're breathing through the nose. The Chinese say that when the mouth is slightly open, all one's troubles fall out.) As always, experiment. Find your own way.

Let's also be very intentional about relaxing the scalp. Many, many of us unconsciously flex the scalp all the time. It's easy to see in a wrinkled forehead (like my own), and probably the same thing is happening all the way around the head. That's a lot of tension, and we don't want it.

And we're not just talking about the muscles; the skull itself is composed of four separate bones whose joints are either in an expanded or constricted state. Medical doctors say the skull joints fuse permanently when we're young. I say conduct your own investigation. Next time you have a headache, sit down and consciously release and expand the joints of the skull. See if it makes a difference.

Have you ever seen the human face in rapture? Just by the way? Next time you run across a copy of *Autobiography of a Yogi*, open to the photo captioned "James Lynn in Samadhi." That, my friend, is the human face in rapture. I've seen photos of death masks that show that same astonishing sublimity. The sight of a face like that touches me more deeply, and shows me more, and teaches me more, than all the world's scriptures combined.

Gazing at such sublime faces, I find it easy to imagine the sight of Prince Gautama on the day his Buddha nature emerged. There's a story about how people approached him that day, filled with timidity and awe, asking, "What *are* you?" They had never seen such a creature. Was he a god? Was he an angel? A devil? The only thing they didn't think to ask was whether he might be a man. No man has a face like that, right? Actually, they were seeing the original face of each of us.

That original face, that astonishing visage of rapture and all-knowing, may come out when we dance, or when we make love, or when we laugh. It may come out when we're doing Tai Chi. And it may not. We're not reaching for it. We're just making ourselves transparent.

Personally I find it nice to know that we don't have to make a face to have one. Once we've dropped our usual tightness patterns, all our various parts heliotrope to their most natural seat of repose, and that certainly includes the features of the face. A new creature reveals itself. Is that creature a god? An angel? A devil? I call that creature our deep organism, and I also call it a stranger because it's a sight most of us have never seen.

The Whole Martial Arts Bit

This book doesn't go into a lot of detail about martial applications of Tai Chi. We do talk a lot about boundaries and assertiveness and how to go about encountering the world. All of that is important work, and if you think you're too spiritually advanced for boundaries and assertiveness, here's a spot of news for you. Spiritual advancement *begins* with boundaries and assertiveness and knowing how to encounter the world day to day.

My martial training is in karate (second-degree black in one style, brown in another), but I can tell you that Tai Chi as a martial art is about being *in touch with*. It's about keeping track of the opponent by establishing and maintaining physical touch. That way, we always know what he's up to and can become the completion of any move he initiates.

I totally get that principle. If I'm out on the street crossing behind a car, I extend one hand and maintain touch until I'm safely past. Horse people do the same thing when crossing close behind a horse, only in that case it's more about notifying the horse. Whatever, when something feels a little chancy, we want to be in touch with that something.

I'm a big proponent of the martial arts because so many of us know practically nothing about taking care of ourselves. My parents' lone instruction in taking care of myself was: never under any circumstances fight. In other words, always surrender to the will of the other. A lot of us get that kind of training, and we wonder why we can't sustain a relationship. Oh, but we're very spiritually *advanced*.

I believe that every child needs to know how to talk in straight lines and how to fight, just as he or she needs to know how to swim and handle fire. It's the basics. Yet most kids are taught to keep their mouths shut and abdicate, and I say that's a huge cop-out by parents who don't want their lives complicated by their children's problems.

It's *not* okay for another kid to steal our lunch money and push us to the ground when we complain about it. It's not okay at all, and for us to tell our kids otherwise does not help them learn how to take care of themselves in life.

First, talking in straight lines.

Kids are basically forbidden to communicate straight across. If Billy sees Susie eating from a bag of potato chips, and Billy's hungry, what does he do? If he's a healthy, straight-across talker, he says, "Can I have one?"

More likely, Billy has been *raised up right*, so instead he puts on a pouty face, stares at the bag, and finally says, "Where did you get those?" Susie, who's reading him correctly, says, "You can't have any." Billy replies, "I don't want any." But he's still hanging around and pouting while Susie finishes the chips. Later in the day, Billy "accidentally" upsets Susie's bicycle and she loses a tooth.

Now here's Billy as a twenty-nine-year-old who never asks his wife for what he wants in bed and cheats on her because she doesn't provide it. Of course, he doesn't get what he wants from outside sources, either, because he doesn't have enough self-esteem to ask for what he wants. Billy's pouty attitude pushes everyone away, and his wife becomes weary of his philandering, so they're divorced before the kids are out of primary school.

If you get my drift.

I used to counsel violent criminals in a group setting, and one of my central themes was learning to talk in straight lines. None of them knew how. None! I remember listening to one guy's hard-luck story about how badly his wife treated him, and I asked, "How do you want her to treat you?"

He looked at me as though he'd never given it a moment's thought. I made him spell out exactly what he wanted from his wife, then I told him to go home and tell her what he'd just told the group. He laughed and said I was out of my mind. I said *yep, and I usually get what I want because I'm not afraid to ask.*

Next class, the guy came in grinning. He said, "I thought you were totally crazy, but I did what you said. I asked her to sit down, and I very calmly told her how much I loved her and what I wanted from her. She couldn't believe it. She kept saying *what's wrong with you? Why you acting this way?* Finally, she shook her head and said *you crazy as hell, but okay.*"

What's so shameful about wanting a potato chip? Really? That's what it comes down to. Shame. The deep-down belief that we aren't worthy of receiving something of value. That's why we never ask. It's also why we can't tell people *no* when we know full well we're being dragged around by our guilt.

Let's be straight shooters. Let's definitely teach our kids to be straight shooters. Let's respect them for demonstrating honesty (unless they're ratting someone out, which is dishonorable). And let's never, ever bait them into lying. Don't demand, "*Who* broke my flower pot?" when you've clearly got murder on your mind. What does it matter who broke it? Get the broom and clean it up. Act like an adult and maybe your kids will be inspired to give it a try.

And then there's fighting.

This will sound strange to you, but by now you know that I don't really care. Kids need to be shown how to inflict pain. How to make a bully back off without injuring him or causing a big stink. Is Mongo Boy pestering you every recess? Give him a dose of pain. Bend his slobbery little finger back until he's begging. Or elbow him hard in the belly. He'll get it. No blood spilled, no parents called, no big stink. It's called taking care of business in an intelligent way.

Of course, kids need to understand boundaries and ethics. They need clarity on when to take affirmative action and when it's smarter to just shrug something off. Yeah, I know, all that's really complicated to explain, but there's a hyphenated word for that kind of really complicated explaining.

Child-rearing.

In the old days of imperial China, every family had its own style of fighting, and everyone was trained in it. If your family was named Li, you were a Li stylist, and that style was for the Lis alone. You didn't show it off to your buds, and you didn't trot it out because someone talked to your girlfriend. No, this stuff was serious and your family came down on you hard for misapplying it.

Further, when you were eight years old, you were taught techniques for eight-year-olds. Nothing really damaging, nothing requiring a lot of strength or athleticism. Just how to get out of a headlock, et cetera. Once you were sixteen or so, you were taught life-and-death techniques.

Today, professional martial arts studios teach the same techniques to all ages. You've got four-year-olds practicing the use of lethal force. That's crazy. You've also got adults practicing techniques that don't match their body types or simply won't work in real situations. That's malpractice.

Oh but don't worry. The whole purpose is family recreation and healthy self-esteem. Right? And operating a profitable business.

And while I'm waxing eloquent, you martial arts instructors might want to take a little interest in what your students are doing outside of class. Have you ever contacted a school principal and said, "Billy and Susie are my students, and here's my number if you ever have a problem with their attitude or behavior"? No? Why not? Is it that you don't know how to use a phone, or do you just not care?

RULE NUMBER ONE

Since we've breached the subject of self-defense, I'd like to introduce the number-one rule of taking care of yourself. It goes like this:

Don't Be There.

When the fight breaks out at Club Rendezvous, be at home watching TV. If it's a dicey neighborhood at night, don't go there at night. If the vibes are weird, leave without saying goodbye. If your boyfriend roughs you up once, don't stick around for twice.

Let someone else have all the fun.

Now you know rule number one.

Here's a bit of lagniappe. We can call it rule number two. When you're out on the street, be alert. I didn't say scared. I didn't say suspicious. Just know who's where and what they're up to. Make early eye contact. Not a lot, just enough for them to see that you're seeing them, enough to demonstrate that you're healthy.

The function of predators is to cull the unhealthy members of the herd. Hate to put it like that, but it's true.

There was one night in Mexico City when I realized I was being followed. I was new in town and didn't really know what kind of scene I was getting myself into. Suddenly there were a lot of unhealthy looking kids standing around and the streetlights were getting farther apart. Instinctively I checked behind me, and I recognized a guy I'd passed a minute before. He was tailing me. I immediately reversed my direction. No subterfuge. No apologies. I just turned and walked the other way. When the guy and I passed each other, he gave me a little smirk. *Okay, you win this one*, it seemed to say.

Know who's around you, and if someone looks a bit dicey, decide where and when you want to encounter him, if at all. The more lights and the more people, the better. Families, especially, are good. Even in broad daylight, I'm not entering a street with nobody around but teenaged boys. I'll take the long way around or else kill some time until a family comes along.

Common sense.

And don't load fear. Fear has a smell, and predators feed off it. I know someone who loads fear and anger every time she's out on the street. The last I heard she'd been mugged four times. Which came first? The attitude or the violence? I don't know, but there's another woman in the same neighborhood who regularly speaks to those same kids when she encounters them, and they share a laugh. She never has a problem.

Before we leave the subject of street smarts, here's a little conversation you may have experienced:

"Excuse me," says a total stranger. "You got a light?"

"No, I don't."

"Okay, great," he says. "You have a great night."

"You, too."

What was that about, that little exchange? Maybe it was someone needing a light. Maybe it wasn't. Most people who have cigarettes also have a light. Don't just track the words of the conversation. Track the body language. People hold themselves differently when they want a light, and when they want a date, and when they want your wallet.

In the above conversation, the real exchange may have been:

"Hey, can I rob you like really easy?"

"Not a chance."

"Cool. Be seeing you."

Personally, I never give a light to a stranger, and neither should you. It's bad for his health, to begin with. And we never want a stranger standing really close while we fumble distractedly in our pockets. Even worse would be to light the stranger's cigarette for him while he steps closer and cups his hands around yours. Keep your hands clear. Never have them in your pockets on the street. If you're shopping, have a backpack and use it.

With panhandlers, same deal. People occasionally need help, yes, but our first consideration is our own safety.

Not too long ago, I lived in a place where panhandlers like to hang around gas stations. They hit you up while you're filling your tank because you can't walk away. I'd see them coming and I'd call out, "What can I do for you?" If they kept walking, I'd say, "Don't walk up on me. I don't know you. What do you want?" I sent them away with nothing because I didn't like the situation. My car was unlocked, the keys were in the ignition, my hands were busy, and there was a flammable liquid spewing about.

Be decisive. Take charge of the situation. We want to be friendly, sure, and we want to be kind, but here's the thing. We don't have to *prove* to people on the street that we're friendly or kind or even half-way nice. That's our personal business. The street is not where we go to establish that.

If you have a soft spot for panhandlers, great. Stash some quarters in a handy, shallow pocket. You want as clean and brief an exchange as possible. Don't be drawn into a huge messy dialogue, and definitely don't let yourself be distracted while a second person steps behind you.

Again, we're not loading fear. We're maintaining a buoyant, people-positive attitude, but at the same time we're taking care of ourselves. That's healthy, and any healthy person will see and acknowledge the wisdom in that.

So, two simple rules of self-defense. Take care of those, and I doubt you'll need a third.

AND THEN THERE'S JOHNNY CASH

Okay, here's the counter-point to everything I just said.

There was a writer (as usual, I can't name him) who took a limo ride with the late Johnny Cash, who was around seventy-five at the time. Cash ordered the driver to pull over for a scruffy-looking hitchhiker. This guy was Mohawked-out and tattooed-out, and the writer felt genuinely uncomfortable, but Cash shook the young man's hand and said, "Where you from, son?" The guy responded very politely. Everything was "yes sir" and "no sir."

A few minutes later, Cash gave the hitchhiker a fifty and bid him adieu. As the limo continued on its way, the writer couldn't help asking, "Mr. Cash, aren't you afraid of picking up someone like that?" Cash said, "I'm not afraid of anybody."

Johnny Cash was a big man. He had enough space inside himself for everyone, and here's the thing. You can't fear someone who's inside you. You'd have to first put that person out, and he would know he's being put out, and there would be consequences to that.

Do you and I have to be Johnny Cash? No, we don't. But maybe we can take a lesson. Maybe one day we're at the park and we have a spontaneous encounter with a stranger with the Mohawk and the facial piercings and the Nazi tattoos, and our first thought is probably to get out of there as quickly as possible. But maybe it's broad daylight and there are plenty of people around, and maybe we decide to remain in the conversation just *one* more beat.

The moment's actually kind of interesting.

We're *feeling* the situation, is the thing. Is there really a danger here? Is this guy sizing us up for some random act of violence, or is he just someone's misunderstood kid in an elaborate disguise? I say we can feel the answer to that question, and we can absolutely trust what we're getting.

"Dude," we might say, "do you know how scary you look?"

God knows what might come back, but if we're coming from a clean, honest vibe, how bad could it be?

Everyone's going through an awkward phase right now. I think Johnny Cash understood that because, well, the majority of his life was an awkward phase. It's tough out there, and patience is always justified, so why not hold that person inside ourselves just *one* more beat and see what comes of it? You never know, but if we're able to hang just a little longer, there may come a moment when Nazi Boy flowers into a shy, deserving human just like ourselves. *Just* like ourselves. Suddenly he's busted and he's grinning and heaven comes down.

Could happen.

Am I saying we take Nazi Boy home and give him the spare bedroom? No, I'm not even sure we let him into the limo. If our body registers the first indication of danger, we aren't even standing there. We're gone. But look—life is over in a flash. We want to remain alert to opportunities to actually encounter someone. We don't want to miss *people*. We don't want to lock ourselves out of a moment that's just this instant about to open wide.

Let's be on the lookout for opportunities to surprise ourselves, to surprise everyone, to remain in the conversation just that *one* extra beat that invites in the miracle.

TWO-NESS AND YOU-NESS

Look in the mirror. I challenge you *not* to notice you're composed of a bunch of twos arranged along a vertical centerline. Go ahead. Try not to see the two eyes, two ears, two nostrils, two arms, and two legs. We also have two kidneys, two lungs, two testes or ovaries, and so on—all of it arranged left and right of a vertical centerline. Even our nervous system is divided into two halves, reporting to either the left or the right brain. Just a coincidence? Sure it is.

Now look at the yin-yang circle. Again we're looking at twoness, and again the arrangement is along a vertical centerline. Again, coincidence?

I find all this twoness fascinating. Biologists see it as a simple exercise in redundancy, and sure, it's great that we have two eyes in case one of them goes wonky—but listen. Our second eye isn't just a spare tire gathering dust in the trunk of the car. We use both eyes all the time.

They work together to give us a far more detailed worldview than either alone could possibly provide, and I think that's probably true of all our paired organs and systems. Even the two nostrils do a delicate, almost unnoticeable dance, alternating periods of dominance and rest. Our two sides work together very intentionally, so let's deflate the spare-tire theory.

A conscious design choice has been made, one that seems alchemical in nature.

We've talked about how, when looking at the yin-yang circle, we can hold our gaze in such a way that the two fishes are seen separately and at the same time unified. With a little patience (try turning the diagram on its side), we see a third creature pop into view. With that in mind, let's return to the mirror and soften our gaze in a way that reveals a left you and a right you—and then a third you that incorporates both.

Focus on the left side of your face and imagine those same features being on both sides. What kind of person would that be? With a little trouble, you can take a camera and Photoshop an exact portrait of that person. Now do the same exercise with the right side of your face. There's a resemblance between the two, certainly, but typically no more so than between two siblings. Both those people live inside your skin. And there's a third you that's limited to neither. The circle of two fishes shows us that.

I say humanness is not accidental. We are pointedly specific creatures. You and I are designed for a purpose, and all we have to do to understand our mission is to examine our design.

Here's a little thought experiment:

Several military guys find themselves airdropped into a jungle with no memory of who they are or what they're supposed to be doing. Once on the ground, they see the plane disappearing in the distance, and they see each other dressed in combat clothing. They're all in great physical condition and armed to the teeth, so they figure they must be on a military mission that required a memory wipe just before they jumped. But what's the mission, they wonder?

They open their backpacks and—here's the money part of our thought experiment—they see what they've been *equipped* to do. They find five days' provisions plus a map and a compass and a photo of a missile-launching site. There's also a big wad of plastic explosives. Obviously, then, they're supposed to use the compass to follow the map to blow up the missile site, and the mission is expected to require five days.

Off they go.

I say it's the same with us. Because the universe is the very far-thest thing from random, we know we've been airdropped here to accomplish something specific. Just as obviously, our mission has required a complete memory wipe. So, what do we do? We see what we've been *equipped* to do. Design reveals function reveals purpose.

You can take it from there. For my own humble part, I see our-selves as having been given a lot of sensory equipment. And I mean a lot. Not only do we have many different senses—all of it arranged left and right, you'll recall—we also have an open aperture to all that sensory data, meaning that most mysterious of all things: con-sciousness.

Elsewhere I argue that consciousness is the one undeniable and irreducible thing. I also contend that consciousness is not closed-cir-cuit but a network. So, the information isn't just sitting there; it's moving in a purposeful way, revealing the universe as being an in-formation-gathering system. One based on twoness.

It follows that you and I have been airdropped to do some seri-ous work in the area of duality resolution. Without a map and com-pass, unfortunately. And with little in the way of plastic explosives.

Personally, I'd say the closest thing to a map we've got is the yin-yang circle. That thing shows us how a triadic system constructed along a vertical centerline goes about the business of cognizing, re-solving, and uploading high-resolution images of probable outcomes in a world such as ours. Look at the thing. See all that red-hot dual-istic energy whirling and begetting and feeding out to the enclosing circle, transforming all the incoming energy into something as yet unimagined.

A good metaphor would be an electric transformer. The reason power companies put transformers on poles goes back to efficiency and maintaining the electricity's proper shape, let's say. If you want the power to travel a really long distance and reach a lot of consum-ers, you have to run it through this special coiled-copper device that keeps the energy in the proper shape. What makes a transformer work? Magnetism. What makes magnetism work? The separation and interaction of positive and negative forces.

Look up "electrical transformer" in Wikipedia and see the various schematics of electrical transformers. Are you reminded at all of the yin-yang circle? Every one of them shows left and right elements arranged around a vertical centerline.

Looks to me that twoness comes here to find oneness through threeness. Our mission, then, may be that of integrating opposing worldviews through the maturation of perspective. Of thine eye becoming single—but not by eliminating the opposing view. When diametrically opposed views willingly reflect one other in a balanced and self-affirming way, the enclosing circle is illuminated and the essential nature of all three transfigured.

And then the mothership lands, and we're all whisked away to Xlandor.

To go back to our metaphor, we now have our map but we still need a compass. What's our compass? I say it's our intuition.

Intuition doesn't get a lot of respect. Call it "gut feel" if that makes you feel better. Call it a hunch. Say you've been consulting your muse. Say you've thrown the *I Ching* sixty-four times in a row. Buy a pendulum and an angel deck and a dowsing rod, then drink *ayahuasca* in the jungle with a barefoot man.

And then do what you should've done in the first place: pick a direction and start moving. Writer William Least Heat Moon said, "Experience is circular. You can't go the wrong way if you go far enough." Just start moving. The samurai used to say that any matter of great importance should be decided within three breaths. Any longer is overthinking it.

It helps to do Tai Chi each morning. It really does. Just as the samurai maintained their razor's-edge intuition through a strict daily practice of sitting *zazen*, we too must lean on our daily practice.

SISTER PRACTICES

Tai Chi works beautifully as a stand-alone practice, but we all hit snags along the way and it can help to come at the problem from a slightly different angle. Personally, had it not been for certain sister practices, I don't know where my Tai Chi would be right now. I've already talked a lot about floor work. I've mentioned Reiki, which supercharged my subtle energy system and heightened my ability to notice it.

Method acting, too, has helped me a lot, as have Holotropic Breathwork, Authentic Movement, Qigong, Healing Touch, Zen, Hatha Yoga, Trance Dance, Ecstatic Dance, Tantra and probably others I'm forgetting.

I'd like to talk a little about a couple of sister practices in particular, beginning with Authentic Movement, which has taught me to become far more honest in my body's presentation. Authentic Movement is a group practice that divides everyone up into two groups: movers and watchers. The movers move; the watchers watch. Then you switch. There's no music, there's no script, and there's nowhere to hide. Someone just says *go*, and you start moving.

When you're a mover, you probably start out feeling very uncomfortable because you're standing there waiting for an impulse of some kind, and meanwhile people are staring. And yet that focused attention is feeding you energy and sharpening your attention and bringing you more and more into the present, and your discomfort may suddenly morph into something very surprising.

Suddenly you're mourning the loss of your mother fourteen years ago, or you're shaking with rage at how disappointed you are in yourself and your life—or maybe it's nothing dramatic at all. You never know. You can't prepare for Authentic Movement, and you can't direct it, and you can't fake it. Authentic Movement is just the goddamn truth, and how could it possibly be anything else? It's coming straight out of your deep organism.

What makes Authentic Movement so powerful, I think, is the witnessing part. I've tried doing AM alone, and it doesn't work. There's no juice. There's nothing on the line.

When there are witnesses, though, each one avowed to be totally nonjudgmental and present with you—you are catapulted into rarified air. You're receiving pure, uncritical, undivided attention, which is in short supply these days. The people you normally have around you? They're busy staring at their phones or at the TV. You don't get undivided attention anymore without pointing a gun at someone, which is one reason it so frequently happens.

We're all attention deprived. We've hungered for it since we were babes and may even have turned our lives into a living hell just for the sake of the attention it's gotten us. Now suddenly it's pouring over us like manna from heaven, and we are fresh-delivered to our humility and our hunger and our honesty, and something emerges that couldn't have emerged any other way.

I've said that the process of Tai Chi is that of responding to impulses rising through the body. I've said our practice is that of assisting those impulses in becoming wholly themselves. Authentic Movement is that process distilled. No footwork to worry about, no choreography to fret over—just pure process. In my experience, it wakes up your Tai Chi like a slap in the mouth.

Tantra training is another practice that can really jump-start your Tai Chi. I say Tai Chi is essentially a form of Tantra. In both we're treading the path less traveled: Vama Chara, the path of immersion in worldly experience. Most spiritual adventurers tread the path of Dakshina Chara, the path of renunciation and withdrawal from the senses. Both are effective, but in ancient Vedic tradition Vama Chara was seen as the more direct route.

There's no reason to fear your own senses. They were given to you by the same benevolent intelligence that gave you a heart and a soul and two kidneys. If it's true that we are spiritual creatures having a human experience, I say let's *have* a human experience. Let's trust the senses we've been given. Let's honor our design to the last detail and see what that may reveal to us.

Out-of-body experiences are great, from what I'm told. But most of us haven't yet had an in-body experience. We're still circling the airport. That's why we are ferociously *in* our bodies in Tai Chi. We're engaging the cornucopia of the moment with every sense we've got, including, as you'll recall, those we don't have names for. If we experience "base" or "crude" sensual enjoyment along the way, we'll probably survive. For a while anyway. It's intention that finally tells the tale. Intention and ethics.

Do as you will, but personally I don't encourage Tai Chi people to investigate transcendental practices that pull you out of the body and put you in some kind of Platonian space. Unless that's calling to you, of course. When something calls, you answer. Just understand that it's calling you in the opposite direction of Tai Chi.

Going back to Tantra, if you have the chance to attend an introductory weekend, you may find it great for your Tai Chi because: number one, it grants group permission to feel. That's really important for Americans, in particular. Every American has a deep strand of Puritanism at his or her core, no matter how emancipated we consider ourselves to be. That strand can't be surgically removed, but we can acknowledge it, and have a sense of humor about it, and overwrite it with a more promising program.

Let's be really clear about this one point before moving on. Puritanism is body-negative and life-negative and Tai Chi-negative, and we want absolutely nothing to do with it. If you feel a pull toward abstention of some kind—I don't care if it's from the West or the East or downtown Hoboken —I say question it carefully, okay? I didn't say don't do it. I said question it. This is the voice of experience. I was celibate for twelve years that I really wish I could have back.

In Tai Chi, everything begins with permission to feel. That's such a big number one that we don't need a number two. If Tantra helps open us up to the body, that's all it really needs to do. And don't worry about finding yourself in the middle of an orgy of some kind; the introductory weekend I attended (Ipsalu Tantra) did not require undressing, and there was no sexual touching at all.

Be warned, though. Your Tai Chi will never be the same.

THOSE DIRTY, DIRTY FISH

Ever *really* look at the yin-yang circle? If you look in just the right way, that circle looks back. There are two eyes, right? The black one and the white one? Always before, I'd seen two fish with one eye each. Then came the moment when I found myself looking at a single creature with two eyes. (It helps if you turn the usual illustration sideways.) That single creature I saw was composed of two creatures whose "eye had become single." Which is to say, their gaze had unified and they'd become more than the sum of their parts.

That's Tantra.

Sorry if I'm belaboring the point, but if we're fortunate enough to experience ecstatic sexual union, our gaze unifies that same way. We lose track of who's who, and what belongs to whom, and who's doing what. We're a tangle of becoming. We're something absolutely new in search of a form to pour itself into. We're a mystery that even *mystery* knows nothing about.

It's the same in Tai Chi. When we hit that sweet spot, solid and empty, masculine and feminine, mover and moved are mirroring each other *so* exactly, while at the same time flipping the polarity, flipping the polarity, we're no longer anything we're capable of talking about.

Watch the yin-yang circle for a while. I say *watch* because there's a lot going on there. Sit in front of one for a few minutes and see what

I mean. I find that it begins to strobe. It's an optical—well, I don't want to say illusion; it's an optical *phenomenon* whereby one can no longer be sure which fish is white with a black eye, and which white with a black eye.

It's like how, when we stare at something for a long time and then close our eyes, we see it in negative. The same thing happens while our eyes remain open. The two fish begin to pop. And the more steady we hold our gaze on the pair of eyes, the more we see. That stuff's not illusion. That's seeing the image as it was intended to be seen.

Notice, too, that the yin-yang circle contains three elements. When the image is rendered correctly (as you'll find in Appendix B), the two fishes are enclosed by an outer circle representing infinity. We've touched on this. The yin-yang circle is not a dual system but a triune one. Again, straight Tantra. Tantric lovers aren't just relating to each other but relating *through* each other to a grand ultimate that includes both of them. That's why it's a spiritual practice.

Again, just watch the circle some time and see what it does. Notice how each fish engages not only the other but the outer circle, as well. Finite and infinite touch, which to me is a representation of mysticism: direct and meaningful contact between a life-form and the cosmic source from which it sprang. No separation. No need for a middle man. No intervening ritual or priesthood required to bring finite and infinite into proper relation.

At the same time, note that neither fish has direct contact with *all* of the infinite but only half. In order to experience all of the all, each fish must go through its partner, as well, through the perfect union of self and self's opposite. Now consciousness is seeing from all three perspectives at once. That's ecstatic spiritual practice. That's Vama Chara. That's a direct path to self-realization.

That's the formula. Embodying very strong yin and very strong yang and bringing the two together in a balanced way that lights up all three perspectives at once.

I've said it before. The yin-yang circle is a schematic illustrating in simplest possible terms how energy moves, which is to say, how consciousness works.

Watch it for a while and see.

THE TWO-DOLLAR TOUR

In Chapter Seventeen, you'll recall, we encountered *the inner glow*, the natural self-luminosity of living things. The inner glow, we learned, is unassociated with religion thus available to everyone, to be basked in and benefitted from in more ways than we're ever likely to know. I'd like to pass along a few other such observations, and we won't stop before elucidating the origin and meaning of existence—which isn't bad for bonus material stuck at the end of a book.

Tai Chi is a threshold practice, a means of stepping from the everyday into realms we might otherwise not have imagined. If we're persistent in our enlightenment practice, and we're soft and absorptive in that practice, one day each of us will cross that threshold.

I recall how, in my first encounter with the inner glow, I sent my awareness to its farthest edge, and there *was* no farthest edge. It went on forever. Then I asked of what substance the glow was composed, and the answer that arrived in me was: *the same thing you're made of*. Consciousness. True enough, there seemed to be no qualitative difference between the glow inside me and that outside me, except that my little bit was *my* little bit. My personal point of contact and my responsibility.

On that and subsequent two-dollar tours, I've come to see the inner glow as a hardwired consciousness network whose purpose is to connect all knowing everywhere with all information everywhere.

Not information in the sense of what's-the-capital-of-Vermont. It's not so much that I suddenly *have the answers*. It's more like I can't find the questions anymore. The sense of incompletion that underlay them has vanished.

When offline, i.e., distracted by the everyday world and the various noises inside my head, I'm still animated by the inner glow—I know it's giving me life—but I don't feel the sense of connection and pleasure that comes with it. Yet the next time I'm able to calm myself down and reconnect—there it is. Every time. Stretching forever, connecting everything.

So, what *is* this thing?

Personally, I find it quite far from random. I'd say someone somewhere is going through an awful lot of trouble. If design reveals function and function, purpose—and it does—I find it hard to doubt that I'm sniffing around the edges of somebody's neural network. God's brain, if you will, or brain-to-be. I'd say it isn't finished yet. Very impressive and very functional, to be sure, but things are still being linked up and synced in and cross-referenced and so forth. There's still work being done.

So here's the question.

What if you and I and every sentient creature everywhere, are bit players in a very large project whose culmination will be (shortly, I hope) the completion of universal mind? Further, what if we, infinitesimally small though we are, have run of the facility? Not just the two-dollar tour. The VIP pass. What if we can log into this network any time we choose and poke around wherever we'd like, for as long as we'd like, and ask whatever questions that may occur to us, and the answers just light up inside us as though they've been there the whole time?

I think that was more than one question.

Anyway, all this carefully laid optical cable certainly suggests a major undertaking of some kind, and I'd say it's centered around consciousness. You and I take consciousness for granted. "Of course we have consciousness. Otherwise, how could we know what we're doing?" But I'm here to tell you that consciousness is not an *of course* type thing. It's highly peculiar, or at least remarkably specific.

It's the one irreducible thing, to begin with. You can argue that the whole universe doesn't exist, but you can't say consciousness doesn't exist. That's why Rene Descartes declared, *"Cogito ergo sum,"* widely translated as "I think, therefore I am," not that thinking has anything to do with it, of course. Nor does "I" for that matter. To me, it's more a case that consciousness is conscious, therefore consciousness is. The point is, we can explain absolutely anything else away as misinterpreted blips on the screen of consciousness, but we're stuck with consciousness itself.

Junior high school science teachers may complain that consciousness can't be weighed or otherwise quantified, therefore it fails the reality test. And I would reply that no scientific observation is possible without consciousness doing the observing, so it's still where the rubber meets the road.

My question is, why *that* and not something else? Consciousness is very, very specific in what it does. So what does consciousness do that nothing else could possibly accomplish? What does its design impel?

My answer would be: it gathers experiences. Consciousness is an open aperture to an experience stream. That suggests that the universe is highly interested in gathering experiences. I'd say the number of conscious creatures lurching about argues that the universe is interested in capturing as many diverse experiences as possible, and from the widest possible variety of perspectives.

Notice I said "capturing." I find it unmistakable that the universe is interested not only in receiving experiences but in preserving them. Salting them away. Analyzing and subsuming them into deeper and broader annals of understanding. Experience is not just a momentary flash of sensory excitement in a grasshopper's brain. It passes *through* the grasshopper and continues to move until subsumed into universal mind. Next question: why would the universe be interested in doing that?

Curiosity, I'd say.

Curious answer, I know, but I'm sticking to it. I say nothing else is capable of explaining the existence of consciousness. Only a very strong primordial pang of curiosity in universal mind could possibly give rise to this vast information-hoarding complex. Why is the universe so curious? Because. That's all we can say, or all I can say. Just because.

Here's a quote that I really like: "The purpose of existence is to make the unknown known through experience." (Kudos to spiritual teacher Almine.)

Curiosity is a unique emotion, as I see it—if emotion is the right word. If you look into other feelings such as anger or sadness, they're easily traceable to a cause. We're angry because of a fender-bender, or we're sad because we've lost an irreplaceable keepsake. Curiosity, on the other hand, has no antecedent. It's just there already, factory-installed, inborn to every last one of us, every creature that draws breath and conceivably those that don't. (How would we know if a rock is conscious?) As I see it, curiosity is as close as we can snuggle to First Cause.

The moment this idea arrived in me, I began to find confirmation everywhere I looked. Show me one child, one kitten, one cub, one chick, one *anything* not wholly animated by curiosity. Show me one scientist, one philosopher, one seeker, one lover, not spurred on by an insatiable desire to experience, to witness, to personally know. Has there ever been a single traveler, explorer, tourist, day-tripper, snooper, peeper, who wasn't impelled by the primal tug of curiosity?

I say, subtract curiosity from being alive and you've pretty much subtracted everything. The more I've observed and reflected, the easier I find it to believe that we are closest to the heart of the creator when we are simply, childishly curious. I don't say that because it's a winning thing to say. I say it because it's the most fundamental impulse we all share. (You might argue that self-preservation is a more fundamental impulse, but I say that only comes into play momentarily when there's a specific need; afterward we return to our usual experience-seeking behavior.)

Of course, you and I have been brought up with the idea of divine omniscience, and, hrrmph, how could an all-knowing god be curious? Not my problem. I don't buy into divine omniscience because that's not what I'm getting. Besides, how would we know whether an intelligence superior to our own is all-knowing? Your poodle probably thinks *you* are all-knowing.

As above, so below. That's what I'm getting. Meaning, both you and your poodle are exact holographic representations of universal mind and so embody its exact attributes. So, if neither you nor your poodle is all-knowing, chances are nobody is.

And yes, I know it's trendy to say we all know everything, it's just a matter of remembering. Whatever. I have to go with my own experiences. When I'm learning how to operate my new phone, I don't say: oh yeah, now I remember. Plus, there are theoretical problems. If we're beginning with consciousness as the most basic thing, we can't say: oh, consciousness exists so we can remember. Wait. Without consciousness, how was it known to begin with? I'd say that's a pretty inelegant way of constructing things.

I say we don't quite get it yet because the universe doesn't quite get it yet.

I don't know about you, but when I look around, I see a lot more wanting to know than knowing. And when I take a really close look at knowing, I see a lot more pretending to know than really knowing. To me, all that's an indication that universal mind is still working on the problem.

I shouldn't say "problem." I see it all as a grand adventure, a hero's journey on a truly cosmic level. The universe *itself* is on a vision quest, and if that's not exciting, I'm sure I don't know what is.

I bring up all this nonsense in a Tai Chi book because that's how the information came to me. It came directly from my Tai Chi practice. When I'm in the zone, stuff just bubbles in me. While that doesn't make it true for you, I'm hoping you may be encouraged to listen really closely to your own nonsense. Your personal truths and your personal practice flow in and out of each other. How can they not?

Those of you who'd like to read a bit more about my TOE (Theory of Everything), proceed immediately to the next section. Both of you. Everyone else can skip ahead.

Let's Say . . .

Let's say one day universal mind was very bored. Bear with me on this. Some truths can only be approached through myth. So here's my myth. Universal mind woke up one day hugely bored because it was in a state of Wu Chi, or unexpressed potential. That's just another way of saying nothing, which was all universal mind had ever experienced. Nothing. Not that this thing *experience* even existed at the time; there was no consciousness to experience it with. That was how damn boring it was.

Not so much as a mouse's footprint had ever emerged from the great and glorious potential of universal mind, and on this particular day that seemed a bit stifling.

"What the Sam Hill am I?"

The question seemed to pop out of nowhere. Indeed it had popped out of nowhere, for nowhere was the only place there was. But suddenly, with that question, one very specific thing stepped forward into being—and that one thing was curiosity. Self-curiosity, to be exact. There was nothing else to be curious about.

Instantly everything changed.

Though universal mind didn't yet know it, its nature was, and is, justice. Meaning any posed question immediately calls forth a completely truthful answer. So when the primordial question appeared in universal mind, it was met by the perfect answer.

Suddenly appeared a magic mirror to gaze into and a pair of beautiful eyes with which to gaze. Either of those alone would have been useless, as I'm sure you realize. Which is to say, consciousness without an experience stream cannot be, just as an experience stream without consciousness cannot be. Together, they provided universal mind with a virtual display that accurately portrayed all that she (works better than he) might conceivably become.

Think of these two, consciousness and the experience stream, as primordial yin and yang, the original pair of complementary opposites. Consciousness, whose nature is to receive, was pure yin; the experience stream, which can only give, was the perfect complement. Together they produced the phenomenon of "the ten thousand things," that is, the vast miscellany of galaxies, planets, and biological creatures appearing as fleeting images in the magic mirror.

The images were not real in themselves; universal mind remained the only reality, and curiosity its only manifestation, its lone step outside the dark recesses of Wu Chi. The dynamic duo of consciousness and the experience stream were the echo of that single step. I suppose you could call all that "real." You can't say the same, however, of the images passing through the magic mirror. The ten thousand things were *maya*, the cosmic dream. Accurate information, yes. Real in and of itself, no.

That's important for you and me to know because everything we see and think about and deal with on a daily basis is maya, an ever-changing virtual display. Which is not to say it's meaningless. It's as purposeful as a sharpened pencil.

The purpose of maya is to portray every possibility, every potentiality lying dormant in Wu Chi. That's a lot of possibilities, as you might imagine. So, in the magic mirror appeared every imaginable and unimaginable thing from a stone to a nimbostratus cloud, from a Nascar race to a supernova, from puppy love to thermonuclear war.

And, very importantly, woven into the whole display was every description of sentient creature, each streaming a running account of personal experiences within the dream. Why so important? Because it wasn't enough for universal mind to read a brief memo: "Congratulations. You're everything that can possibly be."

Not enough. Universal mind had to experience every detail of its every possibility, from every conceivable point of view. So consciousness splintered itself into holographic fragments that dove into the mirror image and interacted with its images—which complicated things more than a little.

Here's where the plot thickens.

Turns out, consciousness doesn't just witness; it deeply affects what is witnessed. In the same way, consciousness is deeply impacted by what it sees. Yin and yang are not static. They are a wild and lusty, freewheeling dance. If we were to animate the circle of two fishes as a video image, it would be in constant flux, spinning, cavorting, warring, swelling, and shrinking in response to each other, yet always meeting exactly. A tempest in a teapot, if you will.

Too, as universal mind saw more and more of itself, it *learned*. Here's where the plot really thickens. As universal mind learned, the eyes through which it saw changed, matured, as did the images in the magic mirror. The whole system evolved into greater and greater congruity, the dots increasingly connected, the neurons more elegantly wired together.

Further, as universal self-knowing became ever more complete, that self-knowing matriculated out to each of its holographic fragments. To put it differently, the sentient creatures within the dream were constantly online with universal mind, simultaneously uploading and downloading information and upgrades and patches and what have you. With total real-time connectivity, the whole system bootstrapped itself higher and higher in cosmic understanding.

But the plot was still thickening. There was a revolt of sorts, a cadre of fallen angels, some put it. I'd rather say that some of the bits of consciousness embedded in the dream "lost their minds" in the chaos of their experiences. It was understandable.

Imagine accepting a challenging job as a foreign correspondent in a faraway land where communications are iffy at best. You arrive only to learn that the government is corrupt, the water can't be trusted, and people are eating their young. Not only that. You straightaway succumb to malaria, rendering you delirious for weeks on end.

You've no longer any idea where you are or what you're supposed to be doing, yet you're expected to do it just the same.

Sound like Funsville?

In just such a way, many bits of consciousness accepted assignments in dark places within universal psyche only to become confused, alienated, and disturbed. Their only thread of meaning was their online connection with universal mind, and it was all too easy to lose that thread and succumb to the delirium of a meaningless life in a random and perilous world. Universal mind found itself, for a time, all but incapable of reaching those isolated souls. Thus, the ascent into universal self-knowing was not a uniformly smooth process.

I see ourselves at that point in the story right now. Rapidly ascending yet stuck in agonized resistance. Deeply confused yet clumsily re-connecting with universal mind and drawing a thin stream of sanity to ourselves.

And it's all to the good. Everything works out in the end. As repugnant as it is to hear someone say that, it really is all to the good, every bit of it totally necessary. Every dark corridor and blind alley has to be walked through. Otherwise, the grand thought experiment is inconclusive, the great adventure of self-discovery is incomplete, and that is impossible. It all has to work out in the end because universal mind operates in perfect justice. Every question *is* perfectly answered, and that answer is perfectly received, no matter how messy the process.

So that's my story, and I'm sticking to it. For now. Check with me in a week or so; I may have something better. Myth can only go so far, yet this may be as close as we can come to straight talk about such matters as how consciousness came to be and what we're supposed to be doing with it.

Experience! We're supposed to experience and honestly report our experience. Even if all we can upload to universal mind is our desperation and our loneliness and our confusion—that's what we upload. It's called honest journalism.

And a bit of humility would be nice. Yes, we're intrepid explorers and courageous foreign correspondents reporting from war zones and all that—and we're also incredibly tiny. No one of us alone can shed much light on just this one "reality." And who can say how many other "realities" are out there, each devoted to partially answering one small part of the massive question *what the Sam Hill am I*? And beyond that, who's to say how many other questions might have appeared in universal mind? Could be billions. Or billions of billions.

If I'm crazy, so are quantum theorists. They, too, say that quite likely an infinite number of probable realities exist, each of them awaiting exploration. They suggest that splinters of consciousness are methodically delving into those worlds, flitting about like bees in a flower-strewn meadow, pollinating this one and that one, and then that one over there.

It has to be done. Every time a bit of consciousness enters a probable reality, that reality *lights up* in some important way. It enters a different category of beingness. It's now on the books, a page in the Akashic Records, another puzzle piece falling into place, helping universal mind construct its gigantic self-portrait.

What quantum theory doesn't even attempt, as far as I can tell, is an explanation of how all those probable realities came into being, or semi-being or whatever it is, and what purpose they might serve. It happens that my little bit of conjecture fills that hole quite admirably.

As soon as the question *what the Sam Hill am I* occurred in universal mind, a list of every possible answer popped up. The list took the form of a very considerable stack of slightly differing virtual realities, each displaying another shade of possibility of what Wu Chi might conceivably unfold itself into. That's where the probable realities come from: they're the list. The reason they're patiently waiting in limbo until experienced is: they have no other reason for being. They're there *only* to be experienced, which can only occur by way of consciousness, which. . . .

You see how it all fits together? Not that I thought it up. It was shown to me. If you don't like what I was shown, take your own goddamn two-dollar tour.

TRUST THE GLOW

If there's a central theme in this book, it's just: trust what you're getting. I didn't say trust something really impressive somebody said. Trust what you yourself are getting this moment. Things come to us when we're in the Tai Chi zone, and it's to be trusted. Every word of this book was written from that zone. Does that make it true? It certainly makes it true for me. You're on your own.

My experience says we're all tied into a consciousness network that's absolutely to be trusted. I have personally checked this thing out and it's clean, clean, clean. See for yourself. Connect up and soft-focus and listen in for a few seconds, and your awareness will be alerted to the kind of information that's moving along the net and what kind of emotional charge it has, what kind of energy signature it has, and you *will know* what's what.

Again, all I've gotten every step of the way is: clean, clean, clean. Clean data moving through a clean system. Nothing forced, nothing spun, nothing stolen, nothing hidden. Everything exactly as it appears. Justice, in a word.

I've found that impressive and reassuring.

You hear so much about difficulty and maya and illusion and "the veil" and portal guardians and demonic entities and other such references to a universe that can't be trusted to talk straight with you. I'm not getting that at all. The universe talks really straight and plays absolutely fair. Still we have to understand the process that's going on; we have to understand that understanding itself is a work in progress.

Personally, I find it nice to know that we can't learn any faster than the universe is learning. We can't jump the curve, and that's a comfort to me because it's not all on us as individuals to figure the whole thing out and become little perfected masters all in a row. Thank god it's not on *me* to respond to every situation in life with unconditional love. That's not my job, and honestly it's not even in my vocabulary.

I mean, we put our best foot forward and all that, sure, but it's *our* foot, not someone else's. It needs to come from where we actually are; otherwise, it dirties the experience stream. We need to remember we're foreign correspondents, and the first tenant of journalism is telling it like it is.

I also like knowing that I never experience anything alone. Experience doesn't just come to me; it comes through me, and all sentience everywhere has access to it. I like knowing that nothing that happens to me is personal because my experiences aren't really mine. They're just passing through on their way to higher levels of processing. We aren't here to understand things. We're here to experience things. Understanding occurs on a much higher level than where we work.

Of course, we all *want* to understand because that comes with curiosity, and we're nothing if not intensely curious creatures. But we actually achieve more in the way of understanding just letting the cosmic breeze blow through us. If we're online with the universe more often than not, we're constantly being updated and evolved to higher levels of understanding. Not by figuring it out, but by means of *cosmosis*, just being so open that cosmic truth flows through us.

Our job is very simple really. Feeling it clean and streaming it clean. We're in *this* moment, and we're not spinning how that feels to us. No self-justifying, no projecting, no cognitive distortions of any kind to dirty the content and bog the process of understanding down. Our senses are open and we're feeling everything straight-on. That's our due diligence.

If we can add a dash of humor or kindness to the situation, great. But our mission isn't to be the Lone Ranger, or the Lone Dalai Lama, or any other kind of hero. Our mission begins and ends with our willingness to be here. There's plenty of heroism in that. Just accepting our role in the present situation and feeling the feelings that come with that. Feeling it clean and streaming it clean.

I think due diligence also means checking our inbox like really frequently. As quickly as universal mind gets it, *we* want to get it. That speeds everything along because the more evolved we can become, the cleaner data we can stream, which universal mind is able to unpack ever more effortlessly, and everything ratchets up and ratchets up until—*poof!*—everything everywhere is experiencing everything everywhere experiencing everything everywhere. And then giggling. I assume.

Universal equilibrium of cosmic consciousness. That seems to be where all this is headed. Everything vanishing once more into the original singularity—but an *enlightened* original singularity. One with no more questions. For now, anyway.

Again, T. S. Eliot put it really well: "And the end of all our exploring will be to arrive where we started and know the place for the first time."

To the Bastille!

It was the Buddha who first stood on his chair and said, "It's messed up." Actually, I'm told his words were the Magahdi equivalent of, "The wheel is out of round," which is usually translated: "Life is suffering." I prefer my translation. Anyway I'm glad the Buddha said something. It *is* messed up.

What's specifically messed up is, of course, you and me. When you look at the plant life on this planet, when you look at all the other animals, when you look at the fungi and the rocks and everything else here—things seems to be generally fine.

It's us. It's human cognition that's out of round.

I'd say we're mentally ill, but how would someone as crazy as I even know what that means? There are a lot of helpful recommendations out there, from eating brown rice to repeating magic words. I say we should all maintain a daily practice that keeps us in a state of *cosmosis*, a state of openness to the flow of evolutionary energy. For some, that may be meditation. For others, it may be art. For me, it's Tai Chi.

Practically speaking, not everyone is comfortable doing art, and certainly not everyone is comfortable meditating—but we're all designed to move. Any healthy primate is going to spend the majority of his or her time puttering about, doing one thing or another. If it's about becoming more transparent to our true nature, then why not let that nature flow?

I say stock-stillness is an abstract idea originating in the head, not in nature. Go ahead and sit if you want to—I've certainly done enough of it—as long as you're receiving. As long as you're not so busy pushing the river (doing visualizations, repeating mantras, doing energy locks, et cetera) that you're oblivious to the moment you're in. What we want in our daily practice is a simple, honest method of arriving in the moment—which is a cliché, I know, but all clichés are true.

Whatever practice you're called to is probably perfectly fine, just so long as it doesn't come with a boatload of dogma. Rigid beliefs bog everything down, as do worship and supplication. Who needs them? Let's keep it lean and clean. Let's just keep ourselves open to inflow and let the rest of it take care of itself.

The thing is, we need to be *doing something*. That's why I titled this section "To the Bastille!" We need a revolution in personal responsibility. Look at the mess that's overtaken the world on our watch! It's absolutely unacceptable. And, while we can plug in many different ways, let's begin with the understanding that the highest contribution we can possibly make is to straighten *ourselves* out.

It's not somebody else who's gumming up the works. I know that's always a seductive idea, but our work here is largely finding ways to subtract ourselves from the problem. If we can come even reasonably close to doing that, a field of sanity will begin to form around us, and no one on the planet will be unaffected because you and I are part of a consciousness network that's endlessly self-reflective.

AND FINALLY

Finally, I frequently say that in Tai Chi we're a lot like gardeners. In part we're running the show, but in greater part we're just watching things unfold around us. The gardener doesn't grow the plants. They grow themselves. We're more like alert, kindly bystanders. The jade plant isn't happy in this spot? We escort her to another. This area's not draining very well? We bring along a little sand. In the end, a good gardener is someone who spends a lot of time hanging around the garden noticing.

It happens that you and I cultivate a magnificent garden called the body. I say magnificent because it's an incalculably connective organism that comes with its own power source and guidance system. I say the body is our greater part. I know people talk a lot about the soul, but that's kind of abstract to me. I mean, can you actually use it for anything? The body's what we use for *everything*, and it was set in motion by an intelligence so far beyond our powers of evaluation that—well, just forget it. Again, our part is basically to spend a lot of time hanging around the garden noticing.

Make a commitment to spend some quality time each day in your own lovely garden.

—W. B. B.

ABOUT THE AUTHOR

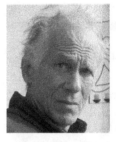 Author William Broughton Burt grew up in Greenville, Mississippi, home to other authors such as Ellen Gilchrist, Shelby Foote, Hodding Carter, William Alexander Percy, and Berne Keating. Burt began writing at age sixteen, honing his craft while working two decades as a broadcast journalist.

Burt attended Mississippi State University, promptly winning a literary scholarship and various awards that brought his work to the attention of established writers such as John Grisham and Padgett Powell. Upon receiving his masters from the University of Memphis, Burt was enlisted to teach English for a year in Shenzhen, China. During that year, the SARS epidemic broke out, and Burt's experiences became the basis of his novel, *The Year of the Hydra*. Burt retired from teaching after a ten-year professorship at the University of Guanajuato in Mexico.

William Broughton Burt's other interests include various martial arts such as Tang Soo Do, Shotokan, and Tai Chi. Burt's non-fiction book, *Tai Chi: Moving at the Speed of Truth*, is his personal explication of the fundamental principles that underly every move and every style of the ancient art.

Burt now writes, teaches Tai Chi, and plays the dulcimer, in the high desert of Mexico.

CONNECT WITH WILLIAM

Fans can write to William at the following addresses:

William Broughton Burt
c/o Grey Gecko Press
38 S. Blue Angel Parkway, Suite 312
Pensacola, FL 32506

wbburt@greygeckopress.com

GREY GECKO PRESS

Thank you for reading this book from Grey Gecko Press, an independent publishing company bringing you great books by your favorite new indie authors.

Be one of the first to hear about new releases from Grey Gecko: visit our website and sign up for our New Release or All-Access email lists. Don't worry: we hate spam, too. You'll only be notified when there's a new release, we'll never share your email with anyone for any reason, and you can unsubscribe at any time.

At our website you can purchase all our titles, including special and autographed editions, preorder upcoming books, and get other great special offers.

And don't forget: all our print editions come with the ebook free!

www.GreyGeckoPress.com

SUPPORT INDIE AUTHORS & SMALL PRESS

If you liked this book, please take a few moments to leave a review on your favorite website, even if it's only a line or two. Reviews make all the difference to indie authors and are one of the best ways you can help support our work.

Reviews on Amazon, GreyGeckoPress.com, GoodReads, or even on your own blog or website all help us to earn more readers just like you and keep publishing great indie books!

http://smarturl.it/review-moving

More from W. B. Burt

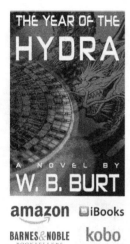

amazon iBooks

BARNES&NOBLE kobo
BOOKSELLERS

books2read.com/hydra

The Year
of the Hydra

Black Rain *meets* Fear & Loathing
in Las Vegas . . . *with aliens.*

"A richly told, diagnosably insane, meand-
ering-yet-captivating journey through everything good and bad about sex, drugs,
and China—plus a wildly improbable tale
about saving the world. In short, not to be
missed."

—*H.C.H. Ritz, author of* **Absence of Mind**

Could a dark agenda be woven into the architecture of China's most sacred ancient temple? An agenda that only Julian Mancer is seeing? Or is Julian off his meds again? If the structure were in fact a doomsday device awaiting an astronomical tripwire—could Julian stop it?

Julian is determined to discover the answer, as soon as he con-cludes a far more pressing matter involving a sixteen-year-old girl with a most intriguing mutation . . .

Recommended Reading

Asperger's on the Inside

"This book is a must read. I adore her style of writing and how open and honest she is with the audience. This book is very relatable and helps me understand my son so much more. Would recommend it to friends and family for sure!"

— *Amazon Reviewer*

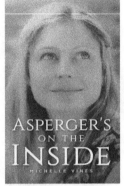

amazon iBooks

BARNES&NOBLE kobo
BOOKSELLERS

books2read.com/aspergers

Asperger's on the Inside is an acutely honest and often highly entertaining memoir by Michelle Vines about life with Asperger's Syndrome. The book follows Michelle in exploring her past and takes the reader with her on her journey to receiving and accepting her diagnosis.

Instead of rehashing widely available Asperger's information, Michelle focuses on discussing the thoughts, feelings and ideas that go along with being an Aspie, giving us a rare peek into what it really feels like to be a person on the spectrum.

A must read for all those who enjoy deep personal stories or have a loved one on the spectrum that they wish to understand better.

Lunch with Charlotte

The true saga of an extraordinary woman, set against the backdrop of history

"*Lunch With Charlotte* is one of the most powerful and moving books I've ever read. Tragedy, loss, heartache... and through it all, dignity and courage. This is a tale not to be missed."

> — *Jason Kristopher, bestselling author of* **The Dying of the Light**

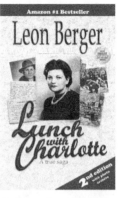

books2read.com/charlotte

Every Friday for the last 25 years of her life, I had lunch with Charlotte and each week she told me more of her extraordinary story. To all appearances, she was a strong and dignified survivor, with old-world courtesies, a twinkling sense of humor, and a lilting Austrian syntax.

Yet deep within, she'd been scarred by a profound personal trauma. Finally, just before she died at the age of 91, she chose to entrust me with this profound secret and all at once I understood how it had affected her entire adult life.

New Second Edition
Now with Photo Archive!

"Mr. Berger transcribes a very emotional interpretation of the events of Mrs. Urban's life. I was moved by Mrs. Urban's ability to adapt to every situation thrown her way. Her life was not easy and continued to be a challenge. Lunch with Charlotte is an inspiring tale and very well worth a read."

—*Heather Robinson,* Readers' Favorite *5-star review*

CPSIA information can be obtained
at www.ICGtesting.com
Printed in the USA
FSHW020319240820
73232FS